The Healthy House Quest

The Healthy House Quest

Finding and Building Housing for Someone with Chemical and Electrical Hypersensitivities

By Jerry Evans

Foreword by
David O. Carpenter, MD

Turquoise Rose Publishing
Snowflake, AZ 85937

www.TurquoiseRosePublishing.com

ISBN 978-1-7334967-0-4

Cover and book design by Turquoise Rose Publishing.
Photos by Dawn Grenier Foster.

Library of Congress Control Number:2019949757

Other books by Jerry Evans:
Chemical and Electrical Hypersensitivity: A Sufferer's Memoir

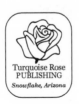

Turquoise Rose
PUBLISHING
Snowflake, Arizona

Dedication

This book is dedicated to Susan Molloy and Bruce McCreary for their contributions to making safe housing possible and affordable to people with environmental illnesses.

It always seems impossible until it's done.
— Nelson Mandela (first black president of South Africa)

This book is sold for informational purposes only. Neither the author nor the publisher will be held liable for the use or misuse of the information contained in this book.

Thank you

So many people have shown me kindness, such as the people who stored my belongings until I had a stable place to live or the neighbors who picked up food in town when I could not go there myself. Some acts of kindness were from strangers, including several medical office receptionists who made it possible to avoid sitting in their waiting rooms.

Thank you to Melissa Allen, Norman Andreassen, Jaqueline Colson, Karlene Coyan, John Crawford, Jeff Crowley, Lenny Dikes, Dr. Peggy Finston, Russell Friend, Tommie Goodwin, Dawn Grenier Foster, Axel H., Connie and Bill Hecht, Randy Humber, Pam Klopfenstein, Bruce McCreary, Susan Molloy, Kim Palmer, Dr. William Rea, Dr. Sherry Rogers, Dr. German Sierra, Deborah Singleton, Jim White, and especially my parents and my brother. I also wish to thank those who helped with this book, including Joy Jaber, Clifton Foster, and the Navajo County libraries.

Table of Contents

Foreword

We have over 82,000 man-made chemicals approved for use in the United States and many naturally occurring chemicals. We also live in a world full of electricity and radiofrequency electromagnetic fields (EMFs). Some people develop severe reactions to chemicals and others develop reactions to EMFs. This response to multiple chemicals is what characterizes the disease, multiple chemical sensitivity (MCS). Those individuals who suffer from MCS, like Mr. Evans, must drastically alter their lifestyle and living arrangements. This book is the life story of Mr. Evans and the extreme measures he was forced to take in order to live a life not constantly made intolerable because of his strong response to a large number of chemicals. But MCS is not only a disease of the immune system resulting from responses to pollen and allergic foods and reflected in sinus infections and elevated antibodies. It is also a disease of the nervous system. In Mr. Evans' case, he developed dizziness and "brain-fog," all relieved by wearing a respirator. These symptoms show how closely related the immune and nervous systems are. As with many patients who suffer from MCS, Mr. Evans also developed electrohypersensitivity (EHS), a distinct disease but one often co-existing with MCS. EHS is a syndrome whereby sensitive individuals develop nervous system symptoms when exposed to electromagnetic fields (EMFs) that arise from sources of electricity and the radiofrequency EMFs associated with WiFi, cell phones and cell towers. There are EMFs generated from computers and automobile

1

engines, and these, things we all take for granted, also cause significant problems for Mr. Evans. The symptoms of EHS are primarily headaches, difficulty sleeping, ringing in the ears, tingling, burning and flushing, and "brain fog." The mechanisms responsible for both MCS and EHS are poorly understood, and there is no very effective treatment beyond avoiding the triggering stimuli. Both of these diseases are increasing in frequency around the world, and increased understanding of both why some people develop these diseases and how to treat them is urgently needed.

David O. Carpenter, M.D.
Director, Institute for Health and the Environment
University at Albany

Introduction by the Author

Having a roof over my head was something I took for granted until I had to flee my home and move to an austere camp for environmental refugees. It was not one of the world's flashpoints I was fleeing, but what most people would consider a comfortable apartment in suburbia. I had acquired severe environmental illness — both chemical and electrical hypersensitivities — which made it impossible for me to live in my home any longer.

The illness drastically changed my life. Within a few years I went from having a comfortable life as an engineer to living on the edge of society and the medical system.

I later moved to the Arizona desert with the hope that if I could find a safe house and escape mold, pollen, air pollution and electrosmog then I might regain my health. It turned out not to be that simple.

Finding a home that does not make us sick is widely thought to be the most pressing issue facing people with severe environmental illness. That issue is the central theme of this book.

This book tells the story of what it was like to settle in the Southwest, the housing options I considered, my living situation and the many challenges I faced. My finances were limited so the house had to be affordable. I could not afford hiring consultants and architects, or indulge in fancy materials. On the other hand, I wanted a house that was energy efficient, comfortable to live in and didn't look like a box of tinfoil. I list the choices I made when constructing my own house, and describe the entire building process such as finding the land, arranging financing, choosing the materials and working with the contractors, suppliers and building inspectors.

I have visited about fifty homes that were built or modified to be a safe haven for people with environmental sensitivities. Some were very nice, some very basic. Some I felt great in, some I could not live in myself. The house I eventually had built was a success because of what I learned from the people who built before me.

It is not necessary to have special skills and knowledge about house construction to read this book. Even though the focus is on the many aspects of making houses safe for people with environmental illnesses, it can simply be read for the human story itself. It may even help convince skeptical friends and family members.

Four acronyms are used throughout this book: MCS, EHS, EI and EMF. There used to be about a dozen names for multiple chemical sensitivity, but today MCS is the dominant term. There are still several terms and acronyms in use for electrical sensitivities, but I have chosen the acronym EHS, which is the one most used by scientists. It stands for "electrical hypersensitivity" or "electromagnetic hypersensitivity."

I use EI (environmental illness) to refer to people who have either MCS, EHS or both. Many also have additional environmental ailments, such as Crohn's, asthma, allergies, irritable bowel syndrome, hyperacusis, light sensitivity, etc.

EMF stands for the electromagnetic field that radiates from power lines, electrical wires, cell towers, cell phones and virtually any kind of electric appliance and electronic gadget.

People's sensitivities to chemicals and electromagnetic fields vary. Many people have mild symptoms and can live a normal life if they just refrain from using some of the most toxic chemicals or use wireless gadgets with some precautions. Other people, such as myself, are much more affected and have to completely alter our lifestyle.

The disease can get worse over time, but doesn't always. If you have the milder version it may not get worse, but it makes sense to take prudent precautions to limit the risk.

This book is a story of hope. It is possible to live a life in dignity and without constant suffering despite having severe chemical and electrical sensitivities. It took time, persistence, acceptance and compromise to get there, but the result was worth it.

Arizona, 2019

The Healthy House Quest

1. Seeking Health in the Southwest

For more than 150 years, the American Southwest has attracted people seeking a healthier climate. By the mid-1870s, books and magazines regularly published glowing reports from people who had found relief from respiratory illnesses such as asthma, emphysema, bronchitis and especially the deadly tuberculosis. These ailments had been known for centuries, but the rapid urbanization and industrialization greatly increased the number of sick people.

The physicians at the time had very little help to offer. They did not understand the origins of illness and could only vaguely talk about "miasma," "vapors," "fogs," and "stenches of rotten decay" as causing disease. They were barely able to distinguish between the different respiratory illnesses, which were sometimes lumped together and referred to as "consumption," though it mostly referred to tuberculosis. Like many poorly understood illnesses, tuberculosis had many alternative names, such as phthisis, long sickness, scrofula, Potter's asthma and King's evil.

As the last Indian wars ended and the railroads laid more track, the Southwest became easier and safer to travel to during the 1880s. The glowing reports of newfound health and the enthusiastic recommendations by physicians convinced many sick people to move to the Southwest. It became a virtual flood of people — by 1890 as much as 20 to 25 percent of the migrants came for health reasons.

Many physicians got sick themselves and also moved. Some recovered enough that they built sanatoria and resorts for affluent patients and they started a society to study why patients got better in the Southwest.

They hoped to find a precise formula for the best environment, so doctors could better advise their patients where to go. Such a formula proved elusive. The researchers agreed that sunshine and dry, fresh air were essential elements and that it was necessary to stay away from the polluted air of large cities. But they could never agree whether high elevations or low elevations were the best, nor could they agree on the best place to live. There were champions of various places, such as Colorado Springs, Santa Fe, Albuquerque, Prescott, Oracle, Tucson, Phoenix and Yuma, which were all unpolluted small towns in those days. San Diego also had its adherents, which puzzled the scientists, since it was a coastal town.

With no agreement on the best place to live, some patients travelled around to see where they felt the best.

With the great influx of people, entrepreneurs soon followed and large health resorts sprung up for the well-heeled patients. Some of these patients were able to manage their businesses back East, as long as they came to these resorts a few times a year.

Since fresh air was so essential, some of the sanatoria were built with oversized porches and large windows to ventilate the interior. Developments of specially designed huts sprung up around Denver, Santa Fe, Albuquerque, Phoenix and Prescott. These rustic huts were essentially screened-in porches, that often had large hinged awnings which shaded the sun when up and provided privacy and protection against the weather when folded down.

The situation for the less affluent tuberculosis patients was much less luxurious. Most arrived alone with nobody to support them, and having spent much of their savings on the railroad ticket. Some people arrived penniless. Some were able to do light work to support themselves, but many became dependent on the overwhelmed charities.

Primitive tent cities sprung up around Tucson, Phoenix, Roswell, Santa Fe and elsewhere, where the sick and poor lived under deplorable conditions. Others ventured out into the desert to camp by themselves or in small groups, where they lived in tents or covered wagons — the travel trailers of the day. Many were ill-prepared for the austere life of the West.

The clean, dry air did wonders for many people. Some became fully well and resumed a normal life. Some people arrived with two years to live, and lived to be a hundred. Many were not so lucky and had to try whatever treatments were available.

Various types of patent medicines, cough syrups, tonics and herbs were sold by physicians and charlatans, but offered little or no relief despite claims of proven effectiveness.

The frontier physicians were more willing to try experimental treatments than their eastern colleagues, in an attempt to help their desperate patients. Some offered treatments with oxygen, ultraviolet light, heroin, rectal injections with hydrogen sulfide and even a pneumothorax machine to collapse a lung so it could rest. There was also a thriving market of faith healers, clairvoyants, phrenologists and various folk remedies.

When some treatment seemed to help a few people, the story quickly sent other patients flocking to try the new "cure."

When the hopes were not fulfilled, people moved on to the next miracle maker.

The world's leading tuberculosis experts met in 1900 and announced that a healthy climate was still the best treatment. By then it was accepted that tuberculosis was caused by a contagious bacteria. People feared infection, so the "lungers," as they were also called, were no longer welcome in the Southwest. Many businesses put up signs prohibiting tuberculars, who now had to live in isolation from the rest of society, and were limited to the company of others with the same illness. Some prominent people said publicly that the Southwest was overwhelmed by the sick people who were an unreasonable burden. Mainstream doctors lost their enthusiasm for sending patients to the Southwest and the migrations lessened. The cure finally arrived in the late 1940s with the invention of antibiotics.

A century later, a similar story is unfolding with environmental illness (EI). Once again, the diseases have many names, physicians do not fully understand the cause of illness and there is no standard cure. Patients can't wait for science to solve the puzzles and have to try a variety of treatments with the hope they are among the lucky ones who are helped.

Some physicians specialize in environmental medicine and offer a set of treatments such as supervised saunas, customized allergy injections and high doses of various supplements, such as glutathione, vitamin C and magnesium. If they do not help, then there are many alternative treatments which have been popular and since faded again. In the early days, these included oxygen, iodine from kelp, injections with one's own urine and the drugs Nootropil and Neurontin. In later years, popular treatments included light deprivation, intravenous antibiotics, hyperbaric oxygen, antioxidants and several types of subtle energy treatments. Faith healing has been popular throughout. Currently, brain retraining is the popular alternative treatment.

Businesses have sprung up to provide better air cleaners, safer personal care products, non-toxic detergents, mold test kits and instruments to measure electromagnetic radiation, but there are also many products which promise more than they can deliver. There are always people happy to take money from those who are desperate.

Like the later tuberculars, people with environmental illness tend to live in isolation or limited to the company of other sick people. Now the reason is to avoid becoming sick from regular people's use of fragrances, laundry products, bug sprays and wireless gadgets, rather than to prevent the spread of disease.

Today we understand that there are many things in the natural environment which can affect people, such as pollen, terpenes, mold, microbes, dust, humidity and elevation. These factors all vary with the location and different people are affected differently.

Many people with environmental sensitivities feel better in the dry climate of the Southwest, but there is no "best place." Some people prefer the hot, low desert in the south, while others prefer the cooler mountains in the north or the very-dry desert in the west. The Southwest is not for everyone, as some people feel better in other regions, such as on the coast or even in places like upstate New York or in the Appalachian Mountains.

Breathing unpolluted air is as important to people with environmental illness as it was to the "lungers." Avoiding noxious fumes from building products, cigarettes, fragrances, fabric softeners and pesticides is consistently rated as the most helpful remedy in patient surveys.

Modern buildings are constructed using a wide variety of unhealthy materials and then they tend to become polluted with mold, electropollution, and the chemical products used by the people living or working there.

The more affluent people can have beautiful homes built entirely of safe and natural materials, while the poor may have to live in cars, tents or trailers. In between are a variety of modified houses and houses constructed using less expensive methods. Old pictures of the tuberculosis huts look remarkably like some used today by the environmentally ill.

Those who are able to move to a healthy house in a climate that agrees with them often see an improvement in their health, though few recover enough to go back to full time jobs.

2. The Road to Arizona

On a cold sunny morning in December 2002 I drove away from the camp. I had delayed my departure for two days until the friendly meteorologist at the weather center promised dry weather and some sunshine for the entire trip. When he asked why I needed the information, I told him I was driving a solar car. He probably thought it was one of those futuristic cars with solar cells all over that some universities were experimenting with.

My car did have a solar panel on the roof, but that was about all it had in common with those experimental cars. My car was born in 1982, and I had modified it so the EMF radiation level around the driver was 5000 times lower than a typical car from the late 1990s. It was a diesel car, so there was no ignition system, and it was produced before electronic fuel injectors and the myriad of other electronics that now fill any modern car. I had then made several modifications, including replacing the alternator with a solar panel to charge the battery. The interior of the car had largely offgassed over the twenty years since the car rolled off the assembly line in Germany. There was no trace of new-car-smell, but a hint of vinyl when the seats were heated by the sun. When I bought the car four months earlier, it smelled a little of cologne, but I was able to remove that by cleaning, ozoning and leaving the car with the windows open day after day in the hot Texas sun. I had to hire someone to cover the interior with a paste of baking soda, then vacuum the dry powder off, then wash it down with non-toxic detergent, then ozone and then do it all over again. But it had worked.

As I headed west on Interstate 20, with the tall buildings of Dallas in the distance, I thought about how I had come to spend 2½ years in an austere camp in Texas, instead of building a career in engineering. After all, I grew up with perfect health — I didn't even get all the childhood illnesses my brother got, and during my six years of college I never missed a day of classes.

I became very interested in engineering technologies as a teenager, especially when I was introduced to a computer in 1976. I graduated with a master's degree in engineering and went to work for a university in Ohio, where I managed networks and computer systems for databases, e-mails and web sites. It was a challenging job that I loved. Like many engineers, I thought technology was the solution to all problems facing society and I enjoyed experimenting with new technologies, reading science fiction stories and the comic strip *Dilbert*. I have used e-mail since 1984, and sometimes became frustrated with how long it took for some colleagues, and the rest of the world, to get on board.

I also loved travelling and have roamed around Asia, Australia, Europe and North Africa with a backpack on my shoulders.

In my early thirties I started to get pollen allergies, which grew worse year by year. I tried all the available drugs, but none worked for more than a few months, except Seldane, which was then taken off the market because of long-term health effects. I was put on weekly allergy shots, which I took for years without seeing much benefit, but the doctors kept promising the shots eventually would help.

In 1995 the spring pollen levels were unusually high in Ohio. On some days I could be outside for only fifteen minutes before I got dizzy. Sometimes it was so bad I could barely stand upright. Before I knew it was the pollen, I staggered into a walk-in clinic and was seen by a physician I had never met before. He treated me with contempt. When I asked if it could be allergies, he replied that everybody thought they had allergies these days. It was just a fad, and I certainly did not have allergies. When I told him my allergist disagreed, he just got upset and left.

I started to get dizzy when attending meetings in a certain building on campus. Someone told me it was a "sick building," a term I had not heard before. This was puzzling me.

My sinuses had been clogged up for some years and now they started to become infected several times a year, each time taking antibiotics to clear up.

I wondered if I could solve my problem by moving to the desert with its low humidity and sparse vegetation. In 1996 I went on vacation to New Mexico, thinking I could find a good job in Albuquerque. I flew in on a Friday evening and rented a car at the airport. It was a new car and the smell of it made me dizzy, but the rental people were very friendly and let me try all their cars. The one that didn't smell bad turned out to be their oldest. I spent the night in a motel room, which had recently been renovated. That did not go well, but I got there so late I toughed it out. It was new to me that new cars and new carpets were such a problem. This trip was a real eye opener.

I spent the week sleeping in my tent and roaming around the different parts of New Mexico. I did not feel good inside the city of Albuquerque. The forested areas in the north were better, but once I drove down to the southern desert my nose and sinuses became clearer than they ever were in Ohio.

I told my allergist about these experiences, but he was not interested and not helpful. I went to various other physicians, even a surgeon, but none were really interested. I switched to an allergist with the highest credentials I could find. His shots made me dizzy and the clinic office gave me a headache, but he said to just keep taking the shots. Then I went on to acupuncture and other alternative treatments. That didn't help either, but at least I was treated with more respect.

Meanwhile, I was steadily losing ground; other people's perfumes and the detergent aisle in the supermarket now made my sinuses burn for a long time. I started getting tunnel vision when I visited my boss's office in another building. I noticed I felt fine when the building was empty on weekends, and also in their big meeting room, which had a separate ventilation system.

My head felt like I both had the flu and had not slept enough at night — symptoms I later learned were aptly named "brain fog." It became clear that what I had was something beyond allergies. My symptoms were much more severe and caused by things that shouldn't cause an allergic reaction. There wasn't much health information on the web in those days, but eventually I found a single brief mention of multiple chemical sensitivity (MCS). From there, I was able to find a few books about it.

Fortunately, my management and the people I worked with were very supportive and made it possible for me to function. I had a private office with concrete walls and a concrete floor, and I also worked part-time from home. My boss scheduled our meetings in a large meeting room with great ventilation, and we arranged the chairs so I could meet with our customers without getting dizzy. When fragrance-emitters became the must-have item for restrooms in the latter part of the 1990s, I was allowed to have one fragrance-free restroom at work. This all helped a lot.

My friends were not into using toxic personal care products, so there were only minor problems there. My hiking buddy used a fragrant shaving cream, but he solved that problem by not shaving before we went on our Sunday hikes.

In 1998 I flew on vacation to northern California. The flight home was full and it was hard to be sealed up inside and breathe the recycled air. I have not been on an airplane since. That fall I spent a week at the clinic of an environmental physician in upstate New York. Finally, a doctor who had a clue what was going on! One of her discoveries was that I was very reactive to the phenol preservative used in the allergy shots that made me dizzy. Other tests documented widespread food allergies and extreme pollen allergies. Another test documented that my liver didn't detoxify correctly.

My health continued to decline and I now had to wear a respirator when I visited my campus office, so I usually went there in the evenings. I also had to buy my groceries at times when there were few other customers, as it was impossible to stand in line next to people wearing fragrances and fabric softener.

After a year, the doctor suggested I get treatment at Dr. William Rea's Environmental Health Center in Dallas. I spent seven weeks there in 1999, which was an amazing experience. Here was a whole community of people just like me, living in specially designed housing, where I felt much better than at home.

The Dallas treatments helped for a few months, but my health declined again during the winter. I was so reactive to ink fumes that I had to read books and magazines on my computer instead.

I started to get a burning sensation in my head that came on each evening and was gone when I woke up the next morning. The burning began to start earlier in the day as the weeks went by, but I noticed it didn't happen on Sundays when I went hiking with a friend. Eventually I realized my computers caused the burning sensation. By then, I would get the symptoms just minutes after turning on the computers. I had become electrically hypersensitive (EHS).

I am not a person who gives up easily. I fought for a month to find a techno-fix to my problems, while still keeping my full-time job going. There were no solutions and hanging on for that extra month cost me dearly in increased sensitivities to the electromagnetic fields (EMFs) coming from all sorts of electronics. Some electronics made my skin burn and my legs feel as if I were standing on a vibrating surface, a phenomenon called paresthesia. I finally gave up when I got chest pains from the freezers in the grocery store and could no longer use a telephone, live in my apartment or drive my car. I had to sleep in a tent in a nearby woods and ask my friends and colleagues for help getting groceries. I was getting by, but I knew this was not a viable situation for long.

It was clear that I could not stay like that in Ohio, so a colleague drove me to a camp for people with severe environmental sensitivities. It was located near the town of Seagoville, Texas, outside the Dallas metro area. The camp consisted of several little steel-and-porcelain huts that people with severe MCS could rent. It looked like a small village out of a post-apocalyptic Mad Max movie. Here lived about a dozen people who had to flee their homes, just like I did. The place was not designed for people with electrical sensitivities, but it was the best option. I could not use the heating system or air conditioner, so it was not comfortable, but I was glad to be there.

I had become an environmental refugee. The term "refugee" usually refers to someone fleeing war and violence by seeking sanctuary in another country, climate refugees who flee drought or rising sea levels, or natural disaster refugees who lose their homes in earthquakes or tsunamis. It seems appropriate as well for people who are forced to flee their homes to avoid bodily harm from toxins, radiation and other environmental factors.

I didn't like the humid climate of East Texas, and longed for the dry, clean air of the desert. I got a directory of intentional communities and contacted some located in rural areas, including a survivalist camp in New Mexico and a nudist community in Arizona, but without transportation I was stuck. When I was finally awarded a disability pension, I again had an income and could work on improving my situation. I bought a carefully selected car model, cleaned it up and modified it. For two years I was only able to get around on the back seat of other people's cars — if the radiation level was low enough. Now I regained the freedom of driving myself. It was a grand day the first time I drove myself to Dallas. Shortly after, I went on a scouting trip to Arizona, to look for a place to live in the desert.

I found five "environmentally safe" houses for rent. Three of them made me sick, one was great but I could not afford the rent. The fifth was a house near the village of Dolan Springs, seventy miles (110 km) southeast of Las Vegas.

Now, three months later, I was moving there. As the hours and miles on Interstate 20 rolled by, I was on my way to what I hoped to be my new home — a place where I could feel better and recover, and have a more comfortable life than what the rustic camp could offer.

On the scouting trip it was still summer, with the days long and the sun high in the sky, which gave plenty of photons for the solar panel on the roof of the car. On this December day, the sun was low and there were a lot of clouds, so the battery was getting flat when I stopped for the first night at a campground in West Texas.

The next morning, I used a battery charger to start out with a full battery. The second day went fine, despite hitting some fog. I was wary of running down the battery by turning on the headlights, so I did that as little as possible.

I was stopped by the police because I didn't have a tag on the front of the car, nor on the back of the little trailer I was towing. The screw holes on the front were unusable on this old car, and I just had a temporary tag for the trailer that didn't look like it would stay in place for the entire trip.

The patrolman was very nice. When he heard that I was leaving Texas permanently, he simply wished me a good journey. I didn't actually know whether my new home would work for me, as it was still being renovated when I saw it three months before. It was possible that I might have to give up and return to Dallas, but I had high hopes.

The rest of the trip was uneventful. As I drove further west it became warmer and more sunny. On the fourth day I arrived in Dolan Springs, where my new landlord met me at the house.

My story up to this point is told in detail in my first book *Chemical and Electrical Hypersensitivity – A Sufferer's Memoir*, which I wrote while living in Dolan Springs. Reading the first book is not necessary for getting full value from this one.

3. Dolan Springs

Dolan Springs is in Mohave County, which is as big as Massachusetts, Connecticut and Rhode Island combined. This huge county stretches from the polygamist town of Colorado City by the Utah state line to the ritzy winter haven of Lake Havasu City, halfway down towards the Mexican border. The county is named after the Mojave Desert, but the county clerk didn't spell the name right, and to this day it is spelled "Mohave."

Kingman became the county seat in 1887. The transfer from the previous county seat, Mineral Park, did not happen peacefully. It was done by a posse from Kingman that raided the Mineral Park town hall at night and carried all the records off to Kingman.

Mohave County is sparsely populated. One can drive for miles in some areas, without seeing a house. Some people live so remotely that UPS doesn't deliver there and they have to travel for miles to pick up their mail.

There is a place on highway 93 named Nothing. There are no houses, just an emergency telephone. The closest towns to Nothing are Bagdad and Wikieup, both more than twenty miles away.

When I applied for my Arizona driver's license, the form asked for my address, and gave me the option of drawing a map if I had no address. Arizona has since made it mandatory that all homes must have a street address, so emergency services can find them.

Dolan Springs was a dusty desert town. It had just one paved road, with no stop signs or traffic lights. There were four bars, five churches, a small grocery store, a bank, a library, a gas station and a few rustic restaurants.

The town wasn't incorporated. It had no mayor and was managed by the county, like any other rural area.

Jeep tours and bus companies came through in the morning with tourists from Las Vegas on day trips to look at the Joshua trees and the Grand Canyon. On the way back, some stopped in Dolan to stock up on snacks and souvenirs.

A local joke was that we had two speed limits: one for the residents and a much higher one for the tourists. Tourists were easy to recognize with their new cars and out-of-state license plates, as they sped through town.

About 1500 people lived in the area. There were three veterans organizations, two of which operated bars. The little library had an active group of supporters, who held book sales and events for children. Two small newsletters circulated, with little of interest besides the occasional bizarre letter to the editor.

Once a year, the town celebrated Dolan Days, with a small parade and various activities. Someone tried to arrange a rodeo, but was not successful.

The Martians landed at Dolan Springs in the 1996 movie *Mars Attacks*, but the producers used another name for the town and Dolan is still waiting for its opportunity for fame.

Land and housing was cheap in Dolan, which attracted a lot of people on a limited income. There were many retired soldiers and blue-collar workers, people with various disabilities, ex-convicts, sex offenders and folks who just wanted to get away from society and be left alone.

People were generally poorly educated and sometimes cheerfully ignorant about many things, but they were very friendly. When I hiked around the area, people often stopped and offered me a ride. When the UPS delivery truck broke down in my neighborhood, it took only five minutes before some guy came out with his tool box and took care of the problem. Another positive was that few people used a lot of fragrances and the smells didn't seem to carry as far in the dry air.

Dolan was a quiet place, with just the occasional drunk driving accident to talk about, like the guy who hit a power pole causing the town to go dark. There were very few jobs around and young people left the area as soon as they could. With little education, the military was a popular way to get out.

It was not uncommon for people to live in a camping trailer and put a small water tank and a garden shed next to it. Some started with an old mobile home, which they built shacks next to as extra rooms. Sometimes the original mobile home eventually ended up inside a full-sized house. There were a lot of ramshackle structures in the area.

The real estate market in Dolan was dead in 2003. Many houses were of such poor quality that they were unsellable and sat empty for years. Houses could be bought for $25,000, but there were few takers.

Arizona is a dry state, as its name suggests. The Dolan area is particularly dry, with only about six inches (150 mm) of rain a year. The ground water is typically 600 ft (200 m) below the surface. Deep wells are expensive; many houses therefore have cisterns and get water from public wells instead. Some people buy a water trailer and haul their own water, while others hire a company to deliver the water with a truck.

A local water company provided water through pipes to the houses in town and some outlying areas. My house was connected to this system, while most of the other people in the EI community lived further out and had to haul water.

The water company normally didn't put chlorine or fluoride in the water, though occasionally they shocked the system with a heavy dose of chlorine so I had trouble taking a shower. When I called to complain about the heavy chlorine smell, they professed not to have done anything. It helped when I installed a chlorine shower filter.

In many parts of the West, the ground water is polluted with arsenic, runoff from mines and chemical wastes from various industries (semiconductors, rocket fuels, military sites, etc.). Dolan had no mining or industry to pollute the water, which comes from a deep aquifer with water that I'm told is 100,000 years old and free from pollution. I just put a filter on the kitchen faucet and had no problems drinking it.

The glitter of Las Vegas was 75 miles (125 km) and half a world away. I could see the sky glow every night, and if there were a couple of clouds positioned just right, I could see the bright lasers reaching upwards from a casino.

Las Vegas was the fastest growing city in the country at this time and it was running out of room. Some developers wanted to put in a 20,000 home subdivision some miles north of Dolan, to serve as a bedroom community for Las Vegas. The authorities required the developer to prove that there was enough ground water to serve all those houses for a hundred years. The subdivision was not built.

We had water shortages every summer. Most houses had swamp coolers, which are cheaper to run than air conditioning, but consume a lot of water. Nobody had lawns, as there wasn't enough water available. The water company signaled their distress level with colored flags to ask people to act responsibly. They also rationed the water available to those who hauled their own water by shutting down the well in town. Water haulers sometimes had to wait in line for hours. This was finally resolved with a new public well south of town.

Deserts are often depicted as flat, dead, desolate places. This place was not. I found the area very beautiful. There were craggy hills and mountains on all sides, with postcard-class sunsets daily, while the Milky Way shined brightly from the star-studded night sky. Tall yucca and Joshua tree plants gave the place an otherworldly character.

The sun shone almost every day. Sometimes I didn't see a cloud for a whole week. Occasionally a single cloud would slowly trundle across the sky on a windless day, and when it passed over the house the ground cooled off enough to create sudden wind gusts as the hot air contracted. Then the cloud moved on and it was still again.

The air was so dry that sometimes I could see rain falling below a cloud, but the rain evaporated before it reached the ground.

The desert appeared dead on hot summer afternoons, with no humans or wildlife moving about. Sometimes I could see a rabbit braving the heat by lying all flat in a small depression, looking as if it was run over by a car, except for its ears sticking straight up. When it started to cool off after sunset, quail, rabbits and humans started to move around again.

The desert is a harsh place, where most plants and animals either bite, sting, carry venom, are poisonous or highly acidic. I encountered rattlesnakes, scorpions, tarantulas, spiders and Wallapai tiger beetles.

One night, I visited the bathroom without turning the light on until I had sat down. Then I looked down and saw two scorpions on the floor, within inches of my bare feet. Note to self: do not go barefoot at night!

Another lesson is to never stick your fingers anywhere you can't see — something nasty may be hiding in there.

I never heard of anyone actually killed by a desert critter. My friend Nevada-Jack was stung by a brown recluse spider that was hiding in his shoe. A doctor had to pull the venom out of the toe so it would not have to be amputated later. The toe hurt for months after, but fully recovered. Another friend was stung by a scorpion. She was sick for three days and then had no further problems.

Dealing with the desert critters became routine, just as city folks get used to rush hour traffic, which to me seems at least as frightening.

Dolan was not a place most people would want to live, but my focus was on getting well and then one has to go where that seems possible and where housing is available. Areas attractive to mainstream people quickly become crowded, expensive and polluted. Dolan didn't offer much to interest mainstream people, but it had a lot to offer health seekers, such as clean air, clean water, low pollen, low mold, no lawns, industry, agriculture or mining. The dry air felt good to my sinuses and made it hard for dust mites and insects to live there. The local utility used an old wiring practice called "delta" that reduces the ambient magnetic radiation more than a hundredfold — my gaussmeter consistently showed 0.001 milligauss (0.1 nT) or less.

The shacks that some people lived in were eyesores, but the landscape was beautiful.

Some people looked at their life in Dolan as an exile and were never happy there. I moved to Dolan with an open mind and the intent to make it my home. That helped me to actually like the place.

4. The Dolan House

When I first saw the house in Dolan Springs, it had just been bought by my future landlord, who wanted to do major renovations to make the house a safe rental for people with both MCS and EHS.

The house had sat empty and closed up for years and the renovations had just started. They had thrown out the carpeting and the wood stove and left the windows open around the clock to air out the place. It was bare inside, with a raw concrete floor, but it still smelled of old wood and furniture polish. (I later learned that the prior owner had a small business refinishing wood furniture.)

The house seemed promising, so I asked to be first in line to try out the house when it was ready. I had arrived at the perfect time, as two other people lined up behind me. I didn't know whether I could really live in the house or not, but it was the best option of the five rentals I saw on my scouting trip. It was time for me to make a bold move and I had a good feeling about it. At least it could get me to Arizona.

It was late September 2002 when I drove back to the Seagoville camp outside Dallas, to wait for the house to be ready. I called the owner every couple of weeks for an update on the project and to be sure I was still first in line.

The renovations took longer than expected. The local laborers did not cost much, but the quality of their work varied. My landlord had to fire the first two tile-setters he hired, and even had to pull up and reinstall all the floor tiles.

Finally, the house was ready in December, and I made the journey there with all my stuff. I had only rented the house for a week, as it is customary in the environmental housing market to try out a place before buying or leasing. It is impossible to know from an overnight visit whether a house is safe enough, as we are worn out by all the exposures from travelling. We need to stay put for some days before we can tell whether a house makes us sick, or at least is better than what we came from.

I tried to sleep inside the first two nights, but that did not go well. I woke up groggy both mornings, despite sleeping in two different bedrooms.

The house had a cement-like smell from the grout around the floor tiles. One of the people from the local EI community came over with a roll of Tu-Tuff polyethylene plastic to cover the floor with, which helped. I was surprised the plastic didn't bother me, but this type of plastic is tolerated by many people with MCS. Another of my new neighbors brought a bottle of non-toxic grout sealer, which is basically sodium silicate, also called water glass.

I slept in my tent for several nights before trying to sleep inside again. This time I tried sleeping in the living room and that worked much better, perhaps just because it was the largest room. I then used the two bedrooms for storage, while keeping the living room as uncluttered as possible.

We moved the refrigerator out to the garage, so I didn't have to be near its electrical motor nor hear the noise. In the garage I used a power strip to turn off the refrigerator when I needed to access it.

The kitchen had an electric stove, but the cooking fumes and the EMF were a problem. I bought a portable hot plate and put it on a table outside the house with a power strip to turn off the power while I tended the pot.

The forced-air heating system was new and bothered me. My landlord lent me a low-EMF electric space heater (now called SoftHeat), but I didn't do too well with that, either.

The bathroom was renovated and had some odor to it, so I kept the window open at all times. It was fine for shorter visits, though it took more than a year before I couldn't smell anything in there.

The house had an attached garage, but I didn't park the car in there as the fumes would travel into the house. I put up a clothesline there instead, to offgas mail, magazines and paper.

Very little furniture came with the house. I first slept on the floor on my old camping mat, but that turned out to be perilous as I woke up some mornings with spider bites trailing across my legs and belly. If that was a problem in January, what might crawl around at night later in the year? Fortunately, someone had an old steel hospital bed for sale. The guy had bought it for his sick wife, and after she died he just wanted to get rid of the bed. He even brought it over on a trailer and just wanted 25 dollars for his trouble. That was my first example of how kind country folks can be.

There was an old wooden table which I didn't like the smell of, so I put it outside on the covered porch, where I used it to offgas groceries. I then bought a glass-and-steel patio table and some simple wooden folding chairs.

Later I bought a small wooden table from a second hand store. I left it outside for some months and it had no smell to it when I took it inside, but it still made my sinuses burn and was permanently banished from the house.

The house was not perfect, but it was a definite improvement in many ways, and I assumed the house would get better over time. Once I was established in my new home,

I slowly learned the history of the house, including how it had been converted.

The house was about twenty years old when my landlord bought it in a real estate auction. He must have spent more than the sale price on converting it into a healthy house.

The original wood stove and swamp cooler were thrown out and replaced with an oversized heat pump. It was great to have such a powerful system that could quickly heat or cool the house, while I went for a walk.

The heat pump was located on the side of the attached garage, as far away from the living space as possible, to avoid noise and EMF. New air ducts were installed in the attic of the house and under the ceiling of the garage, where the heating/cooling unit was placed. They used rigid steel ducts, not the flexible plastic ducts that are impossible to clean.

The heat pump was run at full capacity for several days to bake off the system and the house itself. That must have cost a lot of electricity.

The washer, dryer and water heater were installed in the back of the garage, so they would not bother anyone in the house.

A new electrical panel was installed in the back of the garage to provide electricity to all the main appliances: washer, dryer, water heater, heat pump, stove, refrigerator. All the wiring from this new panel was put in steel conduit to reduce the electrical and magnetic fields. This is expensive work, so it was not done for the lights and regular outlets in the house, except for two outlets in the kitchen.

The old electrical panel was located where the house and the garage met. It was left in place with the old wiring that continued to serve ceiling lights and outlets in the house.

31

The floor was covered with ceramic tile. The wooden baseboards around the walls were removed and replaced with tile as well.

I'm not sure what was done to the walls, but it seems that they were washed down, and just painted a few places with a less-toxic paint.

A few of the original kitchen cabinets were removed, but most were left in place. They were the typical kind made of manufactured wood with a real-wood front. They were twenty years old and the glues had offgassed, though the wood terpenes could still be smelled a little.

All the inside surfaces of the cabinets were covered with "heavy duty" aluminum foil from the grocery store. This worked rather well, though replacing the cabinets with new ones of steel is almost always better.

Some years later, the pipe under the kitchen faucet started to leak a bit — too little for me to notice for awhile. The water collected under the aluminum foil in the cabinet below the sink, where it stayed moist and created a mold colony, so the bottom of the cabinet had to be cut out and discarded. From then on, I kept a little tray under the sink in case of new leaks.

The bathroom was renovated with a new acrylic tub and stall, which worked well for me.

There used to be a propane water heater sitting on the back porch, just outside the bathroom. That was a typical ad-hoc Dolan installation, but doable with the mild winters. I would probably have been fine with it, but it was removed and an electrical water heater was installed in the garage instead.

The roof had old asphalt shingles that were in good condition and were not replaced. New shingles are problematic, and a steel roof is costly.

The house was on a rather small lot of 1¼ acre (½ hectare), which is not much to protect against toxic drift from neighbors. All the adjacent lots were empty and my landlord bought one of them to prevent someone from putting a mobile home on it.

Many of the other EI homeowners in Dolan have also bought adjacent lots to keep a buffer zone from their neighbors.

The house had desert landscaping just as all the neighbors. This was a big plus, since I was too allergic to grass to mow a lawn or even be downwind of a fresh cut lawn. I also appreciated the absence of noisy lawn mowers.

The rent was much higher than what a regular house would rent for in the Dolan area. This premium is common for EI housing, both when buying or renting. It is a small specialty market, with few good houses available and many desperate customers. It also costs more to create a healthy house. If there was no extra cost, healthy construction would be the norm. Carpet over plywood is a lot faster and cheaper than a tile floor. Less-toxic paints and quality materials also cost more.

The owner takes a risk that a healthy house does not turn out well and cannot be rented or sold to sensitive people. Regular people are not willing to pay enough to cover the cost of such a house. It is also not possible just to rent it out to "normies" while it airs out, as they will contaminate it with fragrances, cigarette smoke, laundry products and the many other toxics used in a mainstream household.

If a house doesn't turn out well, the options are to sell it at a loss or let it air out, which can take years.

Several houses that had been built in Dolan for people with MCS had problems and had to sit empty for years. Some of them sat closed up without ventilation so they never offgassed enough that people with MCS could live in them. A closed-up house simply does not offgas.

Some houses that are not quite good enough are advertised for a long time, hoping someone who is not very sensitive will buy it. But people who are not very sensitive rarely move to the remote desert.

Converting an existing house has risks, too. It is impossible to know in advance how it will turn out, though the chances are much better if the house is nearly tolerable to start with. A very toxic house will require extensive renovations, such as replacing the drywall, and may never turn out well anyway.

Some people have simply been lucky to find an older house which has no mold, not needed much upkeep and the people living there were not into the toxic lifestyle, but that is rare.

One conversion house in Dolan took three years to offgas. Then it was one of the very best houses in Arizona.

I have seen nearly fifty EI houses in Arizona and Texas. Some are truly great, but many I could not live in. What will work depends on how sensitive the person is, how much they can afford, and lots of luck. The best houses often sell without being advertised — at least if they are moderately priced.

People who live on Social Security are usually very limited in what they can afford and often have to make do with a marginal house, where they have to keep the windows open much of the time.

5. My First Year in Arizona

The house was pretty good, but still needed some offgassing. This is normal for a recently renovated MCS house. I expected the house to fully offgas over the long summer, where I could have all the windows open the entire time. I just had to get through the short winter.

I'd had tinnitus for years, which sounded like a high-pitched tone, but now I sometimes also "heard" a low hum, as if a big diesel engine was idling outside the house. The house also irritated my sinuses. I had to sleep with the windows cracked open, which worked okay during the unusually mild January. The outside temperature was usually above fifty degrees (10° C) in the daytime and occasionally topped seventy (21° C).

February had more normal weather, with light frost at night, so the house was only fifty degrees (10° C) in the morning. It snowed once, but the half-inch (1 cm) of snow melted away an hour later.

I didn't feel well if I was inside with the forced-air heating system on, so I mostly ran it while I was outside.

I was happy to put up with these inconveniences for a few months until spring arrived. I had spent two full winters in Texas without heat and this house was in many ways a big improvement from that rustic camp.

I went to see an open-air Native American dance festival in February. It was held down by the Colorado River at a much lower elevation. It was so warm down there that all the spectators wore T-shirts.

It started to warm up in March, and I felt better when I could have the windows much more open. I liked the dry desert climate. My sinuses felt much better than they did in Texas and the even more humid states in the East. The dry air made my nose bleed several times during the first months, but it has not been a problem since. I enjoyed that I didn't need to use a towel when washing the dishes and was amazed that my laundry would dry on a line in less than an hour, though I had to use wooden pins as plastic pins did not last long in the fierce sunlight.

There was a small grocery store in Dolan. They did not use pesticides because of the town's MCS population and the air quality inside was so good I rarely needed to use my respirator, but they didn't sell much of what I needed.

I had been on a food rotation diet for four years by then. That meant I could only eat each type of food once per four days — if I ate chicken on Monday, then I could first eat it again on Friday. This is a system to manage food allergies and it has worked very well. I used to be allergic to most common foodstuffs, such as chicken, beef, rice, wheat and potatoes. Now I could eat most of them again and the rotation kept the food allergies at bay.

Such a diet meant that I needed many types of foods to make twelve meals without repeating any ingredient. A regular grocery store does not sell unusual foods such as quinoa, millet, buffalo or ostrich, and I also much preferred organic foods.

Kingman was 35 miles (55 km) to the south, but there was almost no organic food there at the time. There was a big health food store in the Las Vegas suburb of Henderson, but it was a 90 minute drive, which included a winding two-lane mountain road across Hoover Dam.

The first time I drove across Hoover Dam, I nervously eyed the big power lines, which hung so low across the road that they seemed to almost touch the tour buses. It went fine, though.

The second trip across didn't go so well. I got stuck in stop-and-go traffic on the narrow road and had to sit for several minutes right between two big transformer stations. I got so "fried" by the EMF that it took me two weeks to recover.

Some weeks later I got fried again while crossing Hoover Dam. I could not continue doing that. I had to get my shopping needs met without Henderson and Las Vegas. For the next five years, I only crossed the dam about once a year. (A freeway across the gorge opened in 2010, and crossing the river is no longer an EMF hazard.)

A food co-op in Tucson sent a big freezer truck around Arizona once a month and Dolan was one of its drop-off points. They had a lot of great stuff, but almost no produce.

I looked for other options, including two small health food stores in Kingman, one in Bullhead City and one in Fort Mojave, but none of them had much to offer.

An organic co-op in Lake Havasu City then started to deliver organic produce to Kingman every other week. We placed our orders in advance and then drove there to pick them up from the truck. This worked very well, and I got to meet more people that way, too. Unfortunately, there was not enough business to make it economically feasible for the co-op to drive a refrigerated truck the hundred miles to Kingman, so this service ended after some months.

There were four grocery stores in Kingman: Albertson's, Smith's, Bashas' and a small Safeway. The Albertson's store had a little organic produce, so two of us went and met with the produce manager. He agreed to stock more organic vegetables, while we promised to promote his store in our community. That worked well. For the next three years, that store was my main produce supplier. Then a new Safeway store and a Walmart opened and killed off Albertson's, but the new Safeway had much more organic food available.

I went shopping and exploring once a week the first several months in Arizona. I wore a respirator inside the stores, as I had done in Dallas, but now I could really tell my clothes and my hair were contaminated when I took the respirator off again. I had barely noticed that in Dallas, where my head was always "foggy." Once I returned home, showered and put on clean clothes, I was usually fine again.

People didn't seem to pay much attention to my respirator, though I was once followed around an office supply store in Bullhead City by the entire staff. Eventually they nervously asked if I was a terrorist.

By early summer, I reduced the trips to once every ten days. That worked fine with planning and I felt better for it.

Most people in the rural West don't consider driving 35 miles or more for shopping to be a hardship. But it is a change from a big city. I remember talking on the phone with a woman who was considering moving to Arizona. She came from a big city on the east coast and told me she was used to going to Whole Foods every day. She wasn't sure she could live without that. She did move to Arizona, to a place a hundred miles from any big health food store. After some years, I mentioned her concern. She replied, "Did I say that?"

Most people in Dolan had a mailbox at the little post office, as it was very difficult to get on the overburdened mail route. The staff in the post office smoked, which was a problem. We complained to the supervisor in Kingman and he banned smoking inside the post office. That helped a lot, but it didn't endear us to the staff.

Kingman had a hardware store I rarely visited. My respirator didn't filter out cigarette smoke and some of the staff smoked inside. An employee once eyed my respirator suspiciously and asked me if I was one of those people who wanted to take his right to smoke away from him. I didn't know that at the time, but the Arizona legislature was considering a law banning smoking in public places. This was probably what the man was referring to. The law finally passed, which was a great help.

The governor of Arizona, Janet Napolitano, declared May 2003 as MCS Awareness Month. That was a nice gesture she repeated the following years she was governor.

An Arizona activist, Susan Molloy, called me one day and said she was trying to get public funding to build EI housing for people with low income, as people on Social Security can rarely afford any sort of really healthy housing. Now some government people were attending meetings around the state with local charities about housing for disabled people. It would be good if someone showed up each time to raise our voice. I agreed to attend their meeting in Kingman.

The meeting was held at the police station. It was very "electric" there, but they let me speak first and I spoke for five minutes about our situation. One man said he'd expected that someone would show up, as there'd been activists everywhere he went. Not much else was said, and I left.

It took a couple of days to recover from the EMF exposure, which was probably the radio transmitter on the police station. It was worth it though, as four years later, the State of Arizona actually built four houses to rent to people with EI. Of course, that took many, many meetings over many years to accomplish. I just participated in that one meeting. I take my hat off to Susan Molloy who did this year after year and eventually was heard.

A married couple arrived in Dolan to look for a house to buy and make into a safe haven. They lived in a Volkswagen Westfalia camper van, that had a little sign inside proclaiming that the interior cabinets were formaldehyde free. That probably just meant that other toxic glues were used, but the van had offgassed nicely. They stayed for some months at the campground in nearby Chloride, but eventually gave up and went elsewhere.

We had a few people come through town who were looking for safe housing, just as I had myself. About one person settled in Dolan each year I was there.

I drove back to Dallas in the spring to visit the health practitioners there, and did some sightseeing on the way home, which I had not been able to do any of while I lived in Texas. This trip really showed me how much better I felt in the desert.

I did a few camping trips around northern Arizona over the summer, including a weeklong trip to Monument Valley and the natural treasures of southern Utah.

In October there was an enormous wildfire in southern California. It was two hundred miles away, but the thousand square miles that were burning produced a lot of smoke. Dolan was hit by the plume for a few days, where the smoke was as dense as fog. I had to wear a dust mask, while others used wet towels over their faces. Wildfires are common in the Southwest, but this was the worst one I've ever been downwind of.

My landlord hosted a well-attended Thanksgiving party for the EI community, while I hosted a Christmas potluck at my house. I wasn't able to use the electric oven in my house, but someone roasted a turkey and brought it over in an insulated cooler. I could not have a pine tree in my house, but I found a dead cholla cactus that worked very well as a Christmas tree when I hung it on the wall.

My first year in Arizona was the best year I'd had in a long time. I felt much better in the desert than in the humid states in the east. I no longer had to dodge EMF, fragrances, laundry exhaust, pollen, mold and so much else every day. I was no longer feeling spacey and achy all the time.

My health hadn't really improved, but I felt better simply from escaping so many triggers. Living without the tensions of the camp in Texas and having the freedom to drive and explore Arizona also improved my quality of life dramatically.

The year 2003 was a very good one, but that all changed with the new year.

6. Disaster Strikes

The summer is long in Dolan Springs, with a very brief fall. I had to start closing the windows by late November, while the lone cottonwood tree in the yard first dropped its leaves in early December. Winter started around New Year's and lasted about eight weeks.

The house renovations were now a year old and had not been a problem all summer, since the windows were open all the time. I could no longer smell any paint or caulk in the bathroom, nor much of anything else.

Like many people with environmental illnesses, I am the most sensitive during sleep. By Christmas, my sinuses were burning when I woke up in the morning, and it continued to get worse, so in January I had to set up my cot on the front porch. I had bought the cot a few months before in a surplus store in Kingman. It was too new to use inside, but worked fine outside once I covered it with two layers of aluminized "bubble wrap" (Reflectix) that also protected me against the cold. The covered porch was 8 feet (2.4 meters) wide and offered good protection against sun and rain, but it didn't block the wind. I mounted a cotton shower curtain on a metal girder that was next to my bed and that helped with the wind. Later I had a load of concrete blocks delivered from the local hardware store. I stacked the blocks as an L-shaped weather screen around my cot, that worked very well.

It really helped to sleep outside. I had a warm and non-toxic Wiggy sleeping bag, and with the insulation beneath me I was comfortable during the mild winter nights and woke up feeling fine. I spent most of the winter days inside the house, though it made me spacey. I preferred that to being cold.

The house had a heat pump, but I didn't like the smell of the hot dusty air coming out of the vents. It also gave me symptoms very similar to when I am exposed to EMF, which surprised me as the heat pump was fifty feet (12 m) from the living room and the electrical wires did not run any closer. I wondered if the EMF from the electric motor could somehow bounce through the steel air ducts, but much later I realized that the problem was the noise. One clue was that I was fine if I sat on the porch. The thin wooden wall did not shield any EMF, but it dampened the sound.

I solved the problem by going for a walk two or three times a day, while the house heated up.

Forced-air heating systems are not well suited for people with environmental illnesses. Most of the houses in Dolan had low-EMF electric baseboard heaters, but I didn't tolerate any of them, either. Two of the houses had in-floor heating with a boiler in a utility shed, which I liked much better, but that is difficult to install in an existing house.

An MCS friend I had met in Dallas came to visit and thought the house was a bit musty. I tested the house with four mold plates and they all returned from the lab with rather high levels. That was a surprise — mold in the desert? It turns out that mold is a common problem in Arizona houses. Even though the air outside is dry, it is often a lot more humid inside. People tend to keep their houses closed up most of the year and run their air conditioner or heater. With no ventilation, moisture from bathing and cooking builds up inside the house. And, of course, moisture from leaky pipes and roofs can create mold in any climate.

Swamp coolers are used in many Arizona homes, as they are cheaper to run than an air conditioner. A swamp cooler works by evaporating water that is then blown into the house by a big fan, so even though there is great air circulation with a swamp cooler, the inside air becomes very humid.

I checked the house together with the landlord, but we didn't find any visible mold. Of course, it can hide inside the walls or other places that cannot be inspected without tearing the house apart. We did cut a small hole to look inside one wall and didn't find anything there.

I don't know if my problem with the house was mold or something else. It was a converted house, so we don't know the history. There could have been some other contaminants that I couldn't smell, but which I had become sensitized to after several months. I knew I could react to things I could not smell.

I was not terribly concerned. I thought that spring would soon arrive and then there would be another long summer where I could have all the windows open and feel as well as I did the first summer. Unfortunately, that didn't happen this time.

In late January I noticed that my legs felt strangely warm on a long day trip to Kingman and Bullhead City. I recognized it as a typical symptom from EMF exposures, but just ignored it. Some days later, I had the same symptom after a local drive. Each time I drove the car, the symptoms arrived sooner and were more intense. It soon become unbearable and I had to stop driving.

I have had episodes of heightened sensitivities before. Some lasted a couple of weeks, where I needed to be extra careful with exposures, and then it faded away again. I thought that was all it was. A friend brought me some groceries from Kingman, so I could wait it out with no difficulty.

The weeks went by, but the problem did not go away. I still couldn't drive the car, and my sensitivities got worse. Suddenly I could not even tolerate my low-EMF telephone. I had a "tube phone" where the sound travelled to my ear through a long air tube. This system had worked well for a couple of years, but now I could only use it for a couple of minutes.

The social convention for phone calls demands a lot of pleasantries at the start and the end of a phone conversation. They used up the little time I was able to use the phone, and it was impossible to skip them. I resorted to only getting messages via voice mail, where sixty seconds go a long way, and I could check the messages in the morning when I was strongest. I responded back by letter, or sometimes by fax. This worked well for my needs.

Realizing I was stuck for awhile, I reached out to the local EI community, which rallied to help me out. Only one person refused to help, but the others cheerfully made up for it. I knew I would soon wear out my welcome, so I started getting organized for the long haul.

Someone helped me buy a freezer from Sears in Kingman. It was offgassed outside for a few weeks and then placed in the garage. The freezer allowed me to store a lot more food and let me get along with more intermittent deliveries.

A food co-op in Tucson became my main source of food. Their delivery truck came to Dolan once a month, where the local buying groups came to meet it. Our buying group had always distributed the goods among the members right by the truck, which sometimes could be a problem when curious

Dolanites drove right up to us with their smoky cars and stinky cigarettes.

With the new situation, we rethought our system so just one member of our buying group met the delivery truck. He and the driver loaded the boxes into his van and then he drove the load to my house, where the rest of the group waited. I put tables up outside and we distributed the goods undisturbed. This worked very well and turned into a monthly social event.

Some foods I got by mail order, such as dried fruits, beans, nuts and grains from Jaffe Bros. in California. Special breads came from the Francis Simun bakery in Dallas (now closed).

I still needed someone to shop for me in Kingman every few weeks. The co-op only delivered hardy produce, such as carrots, onions and potatoes, and sometimes I needed a book picked up from the bookstore or other errands.

I could hike to the stores in Dolan, but they had very little of what I needed. The bulletin board at the Dolan grocery store listed people looking for odd jobs. I tried hiring some of them to drive to Kingman and shop for me. It was expensive to pay for such a trip, and the shoppers sometimes made poor decisions or lacked initiative locating what I needed.

Then I found a guy who had a small business driving people to Kingman in his van. His customers were elderly or disabled people who needed to shop or see a doctor. He spent a lot of time waiting around in Kingman and could use that time to shop for me.

He came to my house in the morning to pick up my cooler and a detailed shopping list. At the end of the day he came back to deliver the goods. He charged only $25 to do a couple of errands and was very conscientious. This worked out great and soon two other homebound people with EI hired him as well.

He was also available to do taxi service for just one person at a time. Sometimes he even drove people to dentists in Mexico, where dental work is much cheaper. But I was not able to sit anywhere in his van.

A year later, he decided to move to New Mexico, which was a great loss. Then I heard about a company in Phoenix called Boxed Greens. They ship fresh produce in insulated boxes with an ice pack and it arrives the next day with regular shipping. This worked very well.

A few times a year I got a ride with someone going to Kingman or Bullhead City. It was a real treat to see something different. There were only a few vehicles I could tolerate, even when I sat in the back seat. A few times someone drove me in my own car with me sitting in the back seat.

Despite being stuck, I tried to make the best of the situation and was still able to have a social life. I made friends with a retired miner in the neighborhood and three EI houses were within hiking distance. My house was close to the main road, making it convenient for people to stop by on their way to town.

I even had out-of-town family and friends come to visit. One time three women with MCS came up from Tucson. We all slept on my porch and since we all had different diets, we had to set up a large outdoor kitchen with so many hot plates that the breakers became overloaded. I hosted a big party for them where nearly everyone in the EI community showed up.

I hosted various community gatherings throughout the year. These were both holiday potlucks and what we called "sunset parties." The sunset parties started at sunset, where we shared snacks while watching the evening glow. It was simply too hot to enjoy the outdoors earlier in the day. We were typically five or six people for these gatherings.

Despite these efforts I was alone for days at a time. I do like the quietness of my own company, though a whole week without hearing another voice was too long.

I loved books and magazines, but the ink fumes limited how much I could read. At night I sometimes walked around in my memory and revisited places I've been, such as London, Paris, Copenhagen and even my old school buildings. Sometimes I played what-if games, imagining how other life choices might have played out, such as when I considered working in Australia.

Sleeping on the porch was sometimes a bit of an adventure. One night I was awakened by a pack of coyotes howling in my front yard. Another night I was visited by a group of free-range cows that wanted to eat the leaves off my lone cottonwood tree.

I had to watch my steps carefully on fall evenings, when the air was cool enough to entice scorpions and snakes to visit the sun-warmed concrete porch. It was then almost daily I saw a scorpion there. I never had any such visitors on my cot, so it wasn't a real problem, once I got used to the idea of what might roam around under my cot at night. A friend once slept on the ground for six years around Dolan Springs, until he was able to buy a house. He did not have a cot or a tent to keep any critters out, but just a camping mat and a sleeping bag on top of a shipping pallet. He was bitten only once, which was extremely painful for two weeks. This seems amazing, though that was how the cowboys and other travelers slept in the old days.

At least I didn't need any mosquito netting, as very few flying insects could live in the dry desert.

It was pleasant to sleep outside during much of the year, though it was too hot in the summer when the temperature was typically above 90 degrees (32° C) until midnight.

The summer sun was relentless. The sky was clear and blue all day, every day, with rarely any wind. The soil heated up so much that the water coming through the pipes in the ground was hot enough to bathe in.

I enjoyed the heat the first summer, but the second summer my health had declined and now the heat made me dizzy. I had to stay on my cot much of the day, drinking lots of cool water from the fridge and misting myself with a spray bottle.

I went for a hike every morning before sunrise and then did chores before it got too hot. Twice a week I hiked to the Dolan post office to pick up my mail. I did this well after sunset, though it was still too hot and the staff regularly washed the floor after hours, using a horrible cleaning agent. Eventually I was able to get a slot on the overburdened mail delivery route, with the help of a letter from my doctor, and then I only had to walk a couple hundred yards to my mailbox.

I started writing my first book. It took about three years for the rough draft to be finished, as I only worked on it when my mind was free of cobwebs, which wasn't often.

Life was still fairly comfortable and I had what I needed, but I was stuck. The first several months I simply expected I needed to wait it out, that I would get better on my own, especially with the warmer weather. But it didn't happen. I needed to do something more proactive.

I knew it would be a total waste to go to any regular physician. There was one environmental physician in Las Vegas at the time, but her clinic was right next to a big cell tower. I was also told that all the mandatory testing up front would be costly — and probably duplicating what had already been done. Instead, I did phone consultations with Dr. Rea back in Dallas.

We did some lab tests, but I had to go to either Bullhead City or Las Vegas to have the blood drawn. Someone volunteered to drive me in the back of her pickup truck, but the lab botched one test so I had to go back again. The lab botched it again. Then I gave up.

I tried three alternative health practitioners, but none of them were of much help.

I tried several supplements on my own. One was from a company which made custom mixes of vitamins and minerals, based on a blood test. I took the mix every day for some weeks, but then became too reactive to it and had to give up. I tried a similar product from another company, with the same result. They both came as a liquid, so I wonder if the problem was the preservative they used.

Various sources thought specific supplements could help with EHS, such as ginkgo biloba, L-arginine, N-acetyl cysteine, blue-green algae and others, but none of them helped. I had already tried a large number of other supplements over the years.

I heard through the grapevine that sometimes anti-convulsant drugs could help temporarily. I found a physician who was willing to do some experiments, but it didn't help much. I very nearly passed out taking Klonopin, even though I used a very small dose.

I even tried a new drug that was not available in the United States or Canada. I had to mail order it from a British pharmacy, which was legal in those days. (It no longer is, since Canadian pharmacies undercut the U.S. drug industry

— so much for "free trade.") I don't recall the name of the drug, but it too was no help.

Every few years, a new treatment fad comes around. A few people are helped greatly and then many others jump on it. The fad at that time involved using antibiotics for a long time and avoiding sunlight. Some people simply turned nocturnal for the two-year program. This would be very difficult for me, so I decided to wait and see if any of the people in Dolan got well from it, but nobody did.

There were all sorts of devices available with claims that they could make electromagnetic radiation harmless. I was skeptical of these things as they seem to defy known physics, and the explanations offered on how they work were nebulous, unrealistic or nonexistent. I was grasping at straws and finally decided to try one. It came from a colorful catalog that said the development was the life work of a physicist with a Ph.D. They offered small "personal" versions and large "whole house protection" models that looked like pieces of modern art and cost about a thousand dollars. I ordered one of their "personal" versions, which was a pyramid-shaped crystal with some sort of plastic resin on the bottom. The "plastic" was a crucial part of how the device worked, according to the instructions.

The gadget didn't have any effect. I suspect they only work if you believe they will work. The people selling the device seemed to genuinely believe it worked, though they went out of business some years later.

Someone gave me a book about using crystals for healing. I bought a piece of hematite, which is a mineral containing a lot of iron and believed to be protective against EMF if worn in a string around the neck. It, too, did not work. Neither did a few other crystals I tried.

In 2015 a court in Sweden banned the sales of an elaborate and costly device that was supposed to protect an entire house against microwaves, stray electricity and dirty electricity. The inventor claimed it pulled microwaves out of the air and sent them deep into the ground. He was taken to court by the Swedish EHS patient organization which demonstrated that it didn't work and couldn't work. The inventor clearly believed his invention worked, despite no objective evidence, just as there are people who continue working on their perpetual motion machines or other unrealistic ideas.

When the doctors do not have the answers, people experiment on their own. We can't wait for medical science to catch up, especially since there is virtually no funding available. People also experimented during the tuberculosis epidemic (see first chapter) and the movie *Dallas Buyers Club* tells a similar story from the AIDS crisis in the 1980s. In rare cases, people actually do find a treatment, as shown in the movie *Lorenzo's Oil,* but desperate people are easy prey for sellers of snake oil.

During the summer, I started to get a curious tingling in my legs each morning at daybreak. I sometimes get this symptom from EMF exposures, but this was a mystery that only happened for a few minutes every morning. It took two years to figure out what caused it; this turned out to be a crucial piece of information.

7. Technical Experiments

I didn't have any luck improving my health by waiting it out, using food supplements, diet or the few treatments available. Perhaps some technical solutions were possible. I had earlier improved my situation by building a low-EMF tube telephone, and modifying a car made it possible to move to Arizona. Maybe Mr. Engineer could provide another techno-fix.

Having no computer and very little use of a telephone made it much harder to do experiments. It all took a long time.

My first attempt was buying a powerful ozone machine. Ozoning the house seemed to help, but only for about a week each time. I didn't dare use the machine heavily, as I had heard stories about houses that became uninhabitable from too much ozoning.

My car was from 1982, from before electronics became common in cars. It had a diesel engine, so there were no spark plugs or ignition coil. The fuel injectors and pumps were all mechanical. I had already disconnected the alternator and replaced it with a solar panel, as well as other modifications. It was a super-low EMF car, but it wasn't a zero-EMF car.

If I could drive, that would open a lot of possibilities to me, so I put a lot of effort into making the car usable again.

I bought a cheap little AM radio. AM radios are good at picking up some kinds of EMF, which can be heard as static. I moved it around the car, held it up against the wires, relays, etc. There was nothing.

Then I purchased a small probe for my gaussmeter, to see if that could pick up some low-frequency EMF from individual wires — nothing there either.

I didn't find anything wrong with the electrical system in the car. There were no fluttering relays or other failing parts that sent out EMF.

A mechanic had his shop a couple miles away, where he liked to build various contraptions to roam around in the desert with. He was also very helpful and open-minded. He was close enough that I could drive the car over there and hike back. We did several experiments over a year's time.

If you take a magnet and spin it, or just move it in a circle, it puts out EMF. Even a weak refrigerator magnet will affect a gaussmeter that way. There is a lot of steel that moves in a car and steel often becomes magnetized when the part is manufactured.

Magnetization is removed with a degausser. I bought one degausser and built two more myself. I also bought a magnetometer to measure how magnetized a car part was.

First, we degaussed the steel belts in the tires. We had to experiment how to do that right, as the degaussing coil can create magnetic hotspots and make things worse. The key was to turn on the degausser well away from the tire and then slowly move it around in fluid circular motions — never stop, never any abrupt changes of direction. Then slowly move it away again before turning it off.

I had to stand well away while the mechanic used the degausser. When he turned it off I stepped forward to check the tire with the magnetometer.

With the tires degaussed, the EMF levels in the footwell of the car were less when the wheels were turning, but I didn't feel any better driving the car.

Then we looked at the drive train, which on this rear wheel drive car passes down through the middle of the car, very close to the driver. Taking the automatic transmission apart and degaussing the individual parts was not something we could do. Building a giant degausser and putting the entire transmission inside it would be foolhardy, a recipe for disaster, as it is impossible to control the magnetization/de-magnetization of complex parts. It would likely make things worse.

We tried to degauss other moving parts near the driver, such as the torque converter and the drive shaft. I built a big degaussing coil by using a large plastic trash can as a spool. The mechanic slowly pulled the car parts through this large coil and then worked on magnetic hot-spots using the small coil. It was a lot of work and didn't help.

Perhaps a different vehicle would be better? It would be very hard to find anything better than these pre-1986 Mercedes diesel cars. I found someone in Dolan who had an old Volkswagen diesel Rabbit, but it had an electric radiator fan, which measured a whopping 80 milligauss (8 microtesla) in the driver's footwell. The fan could not be stopped or moved.

I briefly looked into specialized drive train parts made of non-magnetic aluminum and even vehicles running on compressed air, but those technologies were not feasible.

Several people suggested I get a horse, but Kingman was simply too far away for day trips on a horse, and I would soon enough get allergic to the hay — maybe even to the horse itself.

Perhaps I could get used to my car by desensitizing myself. Allergy shots work that way — maybe I could do the same. I designed a three-week program to see.

The first days I just sat in the car for an hour, without the engine even being on — no problem, of course.

Then I turned on the engine each day and just let it idle while I sat there. I had minor symptoms from just that.

After some days of sitting with the engine idling, I drove it a couple hundred yards down the road and back again each day. That was okay.

I extended the trips very slowly. I could feel the car, but it didn't cause the burning sensation I expected. It looked like I was on to something.

After the three weeks, I was able to drive about five miles away and back again. I seemed to be ready. Then I had a day I felt good and drove the eight miles to a little souvenir shop out on highway 93, just to have a goal. I stopped there, looked at the stuff a bit, and was okay. Alright, let's test this further. I then drove south on highway 93 to the little town of Chloride. It's a former mining town that is now an artist community. That was too much. I knew I was in trouble when I got there. I hiked around the little town for a couple of hours looking at the artwork displays in people's yards, while giving my body a rest from the car.

The burning sensations did simmer down some and I was able to do the half-hour drive back to Dolan, but it was not good. It took me weeks to recover from that trip.

Desensitization was not what I needed. It could only help a little. I could drive to Dolan from the house, but that was about all I could do and I preferred to hike down there anyway. Maybe I needed to take some other loads off my body. I was right about that, but I kept looking in the wrong directions.

I still had problems with the phone, where I could only retrieve voice mails and not have any conversations except with the very few people who understood that sixty seconds really means sixty seconds. I was strongest in the morning, so that is when I used the phone.

One day I put my cheap little AM radio up against the phone cord. I could hear a lot of static. That meant high-frequency signals were travelling on the phone line and into the house, with the phone line acting as a radiating antenna. I installed a filter and some ferrites on the line where it entered the house and there was no more static on the AM radio, but I didn't tolerate the phone any better.

My problem with the phone was probably the sound quality, but it was years later that I understood that was even possible, and that the sound of the car engine could also be a problem.

There was a big hill nearly a mile from the house. On top were a few antennas that looked like cell phone and television transmitters. About a year after I moved in, I watched someone struggle to get a big truck up the very steep access road. Perhaps they upgraded the transmitters then? My car problems started a couple of months after that truck went up there.

Radio-frequency meters started to become available at that time, so I bought one. I could see that the radiation got lower as I walked further away from that hill. Maybe I should try staying away from that hill for a few days and see if that helped? If I could have used my car, it would have been so easy to just go camping somewhere for a week, but now it had to be close by. I discovered a dirt road going behind a ridge about 1½ miles away, and on public land. That would give me more distance and the ridge would shield the transmitter signals. On top of the low ridge I measured the microwave radiation to be $1 \mu W/m^2$. When I walked behind the ridge the level dropped to $0.2 \mu W/m^2$ or about 200 times less than at the house.

I drove my car there and camped for two nights. It was beastly hot, with the car being the only shade available. The car did not feel any better driving home — another fiasco.

Then I tried sleeping in a Faraday cage. I bought some shielding fabric made of polyester threads with a very thin coating of copper. It stunk so I had to wash it several times, but it was still only usable outside. I hung the fabric over my bed and tucked it under me, so I was surrounded on all sides. I tried connecting the shield to a separate ground rod — not the house ground, which should not be used for this purpose. The Faraday canopy did not seem to help any, whether it was grounded or not. Much later I used an RF meter to test how much the fabric actually shielded and it was very little. Washing the fabric probably damaged the thin copper coating and it was a cheap product to start with. I have since seen tests of shielding fabrics and shielding paints, done by the military university in Germany, that documented a great variance in shielding effects. Buyer beware.

I looked at the electrical installation in the house, including the grounding system (i.e. the grounding prong on the electrical outlets). I did a test where I measured the voltage between the house ground and each of two ground rods I put in the soil on different sides of the house. In both cases, the house "ground" was actually 0.85 volts AC above the real ground.

I have since heard of other houses where the "ground" was multiple volts above the real ground. The house ground can also carry a lot of high-frequency transients, called dirty electricity.

I was wondering if the electrical system in the house was a problem. I used very little electricity, so the magnetic field from the wires was very small. Dolan and nearby areas had an unusual wiring system called "delta," that reduces the ambient magnetic radiation about a hundredfold compared to the standard "wye" system, but there was also an electrical field I could measure by connecting myself to a volt meter. That only went away if I disconnected the electricity. I also found out that there was high-frequency dirty electricity on the wires when I held my little AM radio up against the wires. The increased static was obvious. The dirty electricity came in on the wires from the outside, as I had no sources in the house. I don't know where it came from, but it must have been one of the neighbors or it could be arcing somewhere on an electrical pole.

I decided to disconnect the main house from the electrical grid and see if that helped. My freezer, refrigerator, water heater and washing machine were all in the garage and near the electrical panel. I only used the house wiring for the lights and the hot plate, making it easy to disconnect the house.

I was already using the hot plate outside, as cooking odors were a problem. Now I replaced it with a propane camping stove. Gas burners emit nitrogen dioxide, carbon monoxide and formaldehyde, and the hoses and tanks can also leak raw propane when they get worn. I used the stove outside, which has worked very well for many years now, as long as it is out in the open and not under a porch roof.

To replace the lights, I put together a very small solar system with a 20 watt solar panel, a 12 volt RV battery, two small lamps, and a simple no-EMF charge controller.

This solar system gave me a lamp in the bathroom and one in the kitchen. I also bought two propane camping lanterns, which I set up outside so they shined in through the kitchen and living room windows. They put out plenty of light for me to sit and read on the other side of the window.

Taking the main house off the grid seemed to help. I first did this after being stuck for over a year, by which time the situation was already deteriorating. Major action was needed to save the slowly sinking ship.

8. I Need Something Better, But What?

During my first summer in Arizona, I started to think about whether to get my own house. It didn't have any urgency as I felt so great there the first summer. When I started to close the windows around Thanksgiving, I realized the house still wasn't that great and I got more interested in finding something else.

The Arizona desert was clearly the place for me, and I liked Dolan well enough. But few MCS houses I had seen were any better than what I already had.

There were no less than four MCS houses for sale in Dolan at the time. They had all been specially built to be "MCS safe," but the original owners were never able to live in them and neither could I.

I might not have been able to raise the money for one of these houses anyway. A bank would be unlikely to finance a house that costs well above market value, as they could not recoup their money if they had to foreclose.

If I had to get a bank loan, it probably had to be a more conventional setup, such as buying a regular house which I then modified with money from other sources. I had some back pay from the disability agency and my parents could help me some, but it had to be a frugal venture.

Some people have been able to find an older house that wasn't moldy, fragranced, pesticided or recently renovated. Then they moved in, pulled up the carpet, covered some problem spots with aluminum foil, kept the windows open all the time and hoped for the best. This has worked for some

61

people, but I knew I was too sensitive for such a simple conversion.

Most serious conversions I have seen were much more thorough and done without someone living in the house. Contractors and new materials are very difficult to share a house with.

I did not have that luxury. I would have to move to the house soon after I bought it, so I could stop paying rent. Hopefully the mortgage payments would be so small that I had enough money to do renovations. I knew people who had lived in their garage or car while renovating a house and thought I could probably live on the porch or in a tent for the duration.

Renovating and airing out a house would take a lot of time — probably at least a year. It would be a series of projects that each had a start and an end, and I could take a break between each project to save up money and decide on the next task.

I would first focus on getting a bathroom usable as that is the most essential room, and initially it doesn't need to be as safe as a bedroom has to be. Next would be a room to sleep in — which could be any room in the house, including the bathroom. This seemed more manageable than building a whole house.

But it is a gamble to fix up an existing house. It may smell pretty good when visiting, so it "should" air out — but it might not. I knew I was so sensitive to various chemicals that they could greatly affect me, even at so low concentrations that I could not smell them. And what would a house be like on a hot summer day, with a broiling attic and a warm interior? Or how would it be in the winter, when the windows must be closed?

The fact that it took me a year to become sensitized to the house I was renting was disturbing. Was it ever possible for me to live inside *any* house? How to make good choices?

I knew people in Texas who ended up spending an enormous amount of money and effort to renovate their houses before they were good enough. They had to replace all floors, seal some walls by tiling them over, replace all air ducts, install a steel roof and many other expensive tasks. I have visited several converted houses and it was only those with extensive renovations that I felt good in. It seemed to me that it was faster, cheaper and better to build from scratch.

Another problem was that it would be very difficult to find a suitable house in Dolan, as most were built with low quality materials and a lot of people there were smokers. I also wondered if the common use of swamp coolers created a mold hazard.

It was clear to me that whatever I did could not be a failure. Whatever the result — I had to live in it. I could not afford to buy or build something and then let it sit empty for years, like the four houses in Dolan and others I had seen and heard about around the state. I had to do my homework well.

I thought about various alternative building methods, such as rammed earth, straw bale, adobe and earthships, which are all used in the Southwest. I had read about those methods even before I got sick, and on a 1996 vacation trip I visited a subdivision of earthships near Taos, New Mexico.

I doubt the earthships are safe enough, as they have hundreds of used automobile tires embedded in their walls. The tires are covered with stucco, but stucco is porous so the fumes may still get through. Straw bale houses may have a similar problem, as I don't like the smell of straw, and I heard stories where the straw walls got moldy.

Adobe houses seemed enticing, with bricks made of dirt and straw. But then I learned that the builders add asphalt, and sometimes even kerosene, to their bricks to make them stronger and protect against moisture. The traditional additive-free adobe bricks would require major annual maintenance and seemed like a major mold hazard. I later also heard of problems with the grease used on the forms when producing the bricks.

Rammed earth looked more promising. I once visited a rammed earth house near Tucson and liked it very much. It was only a couple of years old and had no odor to it, even on a hot day. Fired bricks and concrete blocks were other possibilities for both the inside and outside walls.

It was intriguing to consider these materials, but the fundamental problem was that these methods were very labor intensive. If I could not do all the heavy work myself, such houses were too costly.

I once read a book with the enticing title *The $50 & Up Underground House Book,* by Mike Oehle, who suggests building buried houses using scrounged materials. Many years ago, I visited underground houses in the deserts of Turkey and Tunisia and even slept in two of them. They were very rustic, but pleasantly cool in the hot summer.

I could see various problems living in such a deep basement, such as rain seepage and outright flooding by the deluges we occasionally get. I would need to insulate and drywall the walls and ceiling, so such a cave-house would still have problems. Oehle advocates saving money by scrounging discarded windows, doors and lumber, but most conventional materials are unhealthy, and recycled materials can be contaminated in many ways.

I was used to apartment living, where electricity, water, sewage and repairs were handled by others. Now I needed to learn about all these things and come up with a plan, so I read various books about conventional construction, and even how to dispose of waste water through composting toilets, graywater systems and sawdust toilets. There was much to learn, and it was slow going as my mind was spaced out much of the time. It was so easy to just let the time roll by. I slowly plugged on, trying to put together a list of materials I could afford and trust.

One day I got a note to talk to the postmaster in Dolan. She handed me a plastic bag with a thick envelope inside and a note from the Postal Service. I had asked a manufacturer to send me a sample of their non-toxic building product, which came as a white powder. They had simply put a handful of the powder into an ordinary envelope that had leaked, causing quite a stir at the Phoenix postal center, which had called in a hazmat response team. The note included a laboratory analysis of the powder, documenting that it was not a hazardous substance.

I became fascinated by Autoclaved Aerated Concrete, which are blocks made of concrete with a lot of tiny air bubbles. This makes them much lighter than the typical concrete blocks, and they insulate so well that in the Dolan climate there would be no need for any additional insulation. The blocks are porous and they absorb water like a sponge, but a special sealer is available, so there is no need for any siding or drywall. These blocks could be a complete wall in themselves.

Walls made of these blocks can be used in climates with warm and humid summers, where the walls must be able to breathe.

The manufacturer in Arizona sent me a sample with the sealer on it. It stunk terribly for a month and then became odorless. I found someone with severe MCS who had recently had a house built of these blocks and she did very well with them. I was able to get several blocks to try out, and I did fine, too. The factory in Arizona has since closed and I have heard of people having problems with another brand of these blocks which arrived oily. Some manufacturers may also add fly ash or mine tailings to their product.

A friend I met in Dallas was interested in moving to the Southwest when her husband retired. She used her computer to check out a lot of small towns, looking for one with a good health food store, no polluting industries and a balanced political scene. Since they were married, it was not important to live in an area with an EI community.

A lot of information can be gleaned from various local newsletters. She sent me interesting printouts about promising towns, such as Bisbee, Flagstaff and Silver City.

I read articles about various forms of intentional communities, where like-minded people live together in neighborhoods. Many of them are organized so a trust owns the land, while the people own the houses on the land. Such a setup makes it affordable to have a large buffer to the toxic world outside.

I have met three people who live in such communities. Everybody there is "green minded," but green is not the same as "EI safe." Burning firewood is considered green, some people use essential oils and other problematic products, and they rarely consider wireless devices a health hazard. Many "green" building products are also problematic for people with MCS, such as various recycled materials and aromatic wood products.

I read about the Dancing Rabbit community in Missouri, where each person has just a tiny one-room hut, while all cooking and bathroom facilities are in shared buildings. The same idea has been used to house homeless people in the Quixote Village in Washington State. These radical approaches dramatically reduce the cost of housing, but my experience living in Texas and elsewhere shows that living that close together does not work well for the environmentally ill. There are too many incompatible sensitivities to share bathrooms and kitchen facilities.

An EI neighborhood seemed to be the best option. It has the benefit of less-toxic neighbors and the option of a social life and mutual support, while avoiding the problems of shared spaces. There have been some attempts at creating such neighborhoods, but few successes. Some have simply evolved with people buying land and building houses next to each other, while others have attempted to buy a large piece of land and sell off individual lots to people who meet certain criteria.

Based on my experience in Dolan and elsewhere, I think a rural neighborhood where each house has 10 acres (4 hectares) is good. More is better. Even a hundred acres does not fully protect a house if directly downwind from a smoky woodstove, or someone burning trash, but the odds improve with size.

Large lots are available and affordable in some rural areas of the American West. Dolan was already subdivided into smaller lots, which increased the price per acre.

9. Remote Basic

I visited a local realtor a month before I became unable to drive. He specialized in undeveloped land and gave me maps and listings I used to look around on my own to get an idea of what was available and what it cost.

I noticed that several of the homes in Dolan had started out as travel trailers, small cabins or single-wide mobile homes, that were then added onto later. That is what poor people do in areas where the building codes are lax. There were no building codes for the Dolan area (there are now), so people could be as creative as they wanted.

Perhaps I could learn from the locals. If I could start small and stop paying the high rent for the MCS house, I could use the money for a real house later.

The camping trailer has a special place in EI lore. The thought of a portable home stirs the imagination with the ability to simply move around until the perfect place is found and if a bad neighbor moves in next door, it is just a matter of hitching up and moving on to new adventures. The reality seldom lives up to this romantic view.

Camping trailers are very small spaces, which only have room for the basic necessities. The small volume of air means that items that are fine in the larger airspace of a house may not be tolerable in a camper. Camping trailers are poorly insulated, so they get very hot in the summer sun and cold on winter nights, even with good heating and cooling. Materials offgas in a hot trailer, and the heating and cooling systems are often difficult to tolerate.

Lightweight materials are used to reduce the weight and cost of the trailer, and the hull has many penetrations for slideouts, windows and vents. Then the sun and rain start working on it, together with the flexing and shaking while rolling down the highway. The result is often a leaky roof, a leaky slideout, leaky pipes, condensation inside the walls and a short lifespan with lots of repairs. Most trailers do not last ten years and by then they are almost all musty inside — a fact sellers often try to hide with fragrances.

I spent several months visiting a large number of RV dealers while I lived near Dallas, and I never found a usable camping trailer. New RVs are built of toxic materials, which are doubly potent in the small airspace. It takes many years to somewhat offgas a new trailer, and most models use vinyl on the walls that never fully offgasses. Used trailers will be contaminated with fragrances, pesticides, laundry chemicals and much else that may take years to offgas, even with the windows open 24/7. And then they almost invariably get musty, unless they've been kept in a garage in a dry climate. Virtually all the trailers I saw in Dallas were musty, and some even had water on the floor after a recent rain shower.

The chances of finding a trailer that is not moldy is better in the desert, but it is still very rare to find a usable camper on a dealer's lot. Any such trailer will need work to make it livable for someone with MCS, and it is impossible to know if such a renovation will be successful. The renovations may cost more than the purchase price.

I have seen several attempts at low-cost renovations, where the camper was stripped to the outer walls, with cabinets, inner walls, and insulation removed with only the floor, outer walls and studs left. Such a trailer is just a bare room on wheels, without any amenities. And still they smelled to me, especially the old wooden studs. I don't know anyone who actually lived in one of those stripped trailers.

A few premium campers are built to last, such as Airstream, Avion and perhaps CampLite, but they also cost a lot more. The Airstreams are built like the hull of an aircraft making them much more durable and less likely to leak, but they are still prone to condensation inside the wall cavities, so the insulation gets wet and moldy. Airstream trailers from the 1950s and 1960s have been used by many people with MCS. They generally need extensive renovations, such as dismantling the inner walls, replacing the moldy insulation, cabinets, floor, etc. It is a large project and people who have done it all told me they did not want to do it again.

In the late 1960s Airstream started to coat their inner walls with vinyl, which never offgasses. There was one of those in the Seagoville camp. The owners had tried to seal the curved vinyl walls by fully covering them with aluminum tape. It took an amazing number of rolls. Even a decade later that camper still smelled of the tape-glue on hot days. It never became habitable.

I have visited a radically renovated Airstream, where everything inside was replaced with aluminum plates and stainless steel: floor, dividing walls, cabinets, kitchen counter, shower stall, etc. It had a strong metallic odor I could not live with. I think they used raw aluminum plates instead of anodized aluminum.

There are people who specialize in renovating old trailers for people with MCS. I don't think I have ever seen any of their trailers.

Some people have tried to simply find a less-moldy camper from a desert area, then wash it down, cover the floor with a membrane and loose porcelain tiles, remove most of the furniture and cabinets and seal the rest. Then they air it out for a long time with the windows open all day. This all helped a lot, though even a year later it was not that great.

I have visited about two dozen MCS camping trailers and I doubt I could live well in any of them. Most had some odor to them, and many of them also gave me EMF-type symptoms, which I'm not sure why, as some had no electricity in or near them at all. I seem to have a problem with metal floors, so perhaps being inside a small metallic room was the problem, though I feel fine in houses with metal roofs and siding.

The closest to perfection I have seen was a porcelain trailer in pristine condition. It was built by Dr. Mike Lattieri and owned by the late singer-songwriter Kim Palmer. Kim produced the album *Songs from a porcelain trailer* while living in this trailer on top of a mesa in Arizona. Dr. Lattieri has built many trailers and portable huts of porcelainized steel, but he no longer does.

More recently has come the tiny house movement. This is a variation of the travel trailer setup with a tiny cabin built on wheels. Building them of healthy materials tends to be costly if you can't do the work yourself and the weight limitations make it necessary to compromise with the materials. It has been done, but with a lot of interior wood and limited insulation.

Converting a mobile home is another option. New mobile homes are too toxic to convert, but I've seen two renovated used ones. In both cases they had been well maintained and had no leaks or mold. One of them had never been sprayed either. For that one, the new owner sealed all the walls, ceilings and cabinets with aluminum foil. The floor was covered with galvanized steel plates. When it was finished it had no smell that I could detect, but the owner was able to be

71

there in the daytime only. She could not sleep there at night and ended up renting it out to two people with MCS who both felt well there.

The other mobile home I've seen was stripped to the outside walls and roof. It was then rebuilt with healthier materials. This work cost nearly $80,000. Then came the cost of buying the mobile home and a lot with well, sewage and electricity. For little extra money one could have a site-built house with radiant-floor heating, better materials and a property that increases in value over time. At least the owner was able to live in it, though he did buy a real house some years later.

I looked into yurts, which are round tent houses with semi-solid walls. They were invented by Mongol nomads and are available in modern versions. They are mostly used as vacation homes, but can be used for full-time living. I have been inside a yurt that stunk like a tent, which is not surprising as the materials are very similar.

I have also visited a large geodesic dome tent house, which had some sort of plastic over a steel frame. Despite the large airspace, there was still a plastic smell inside, though less than inside a tent.

Regular tents are made of polyester or nylon and treated with herbicides, flame retardants, UV protectors, etc. The plastic does not last without these chemicals. I had a tent that took two years to offgas enough to be usable at night. Even after using it for years, it still smelled when sitting in the sun.

I found a company which makes tents of cotton. They sell teepees and various tents used in medieval festivals and Civil War reenactments. They even offered tents of untreated cotton. I visited someone who lived in such a tent — even in dry Arizona it was black with mold after a year or two.

It was clear to me that I needed housing built of solid materials. Nothing portable seemed realistic.

The shacks I saw around Dolan, and some rustic EI living situations I've seen, inspired me to think up something that could work. It consisted of three structures: one was a fully heated and insulated one-room hut of about 12x12 feet (4x4 meters), that would be my living room and bedroom.

The hut could be built with the autoclaved aerated concrete blocks I had found, with steel plates as ceiling, and a steel roof. The floor could be patio pavers on light gravel. No need for any toxic paint or drywall.

If I decided on radiant floor heating, I could bury insulating foam boards in the sand under the patio pavers and install PEX pipes between the pavers and the insulation. Or the floor could be an insulated concrete slab, which could be buffed and sealed to look good.

There would also be two sheds next to the hut. One shed would have the kitchen, shower and toilet, the other all the mechanical things I wanted some distance from, such as water heater, refrigerator, water pump, etc. These two sheds would be simple steel garden sheds, with aluminized "bubble wrap" insulation.

Between my living hut and the kitchen hut would be a large ramada shade structure, so I could be outside much of the day. Then it would not matter much that my indoor living space was so small.

The kitchen and living huts would be heated with radiators or in-floor heating, with the hot water coming from a boiler in the utility shed.

I didn't know of any way to cool the place that I could tolerate. I didn't like the noise and EMF from air conditioners. Swamp coolers also had these problems, besides mold issues. An alternative is to cool the air by pulling it through deeply buried air tubes, but they tend to have problems with condensation and mold. I thought I could make do without cooling, just as people used to in the old days.

I considered simply buying a cheap old camping trailer for $1,000 and using that as the bathroom, but cheap old trailers are very moldy. I knew from experience that even a short visit inside would make my hair and clothes smell moldy.

I called the county health department who told me they saw no problem if I used a composting toilet, but I still had to have a septic system for the kitchen sink. (I didn't ask what they thought about a sawdust toilet.) I thought I could install a composting toilet and use a graywater system for the sink until someone complained. Several years later I talked to two owners of composting toilets who both told me these toilets are fussy and require a lot of maintenance to be odorless.

Since I would be outside most of the day, I needed very clean outside air. That meant distance from any neighbors. Dolan lots were all 1¼ acres (0.5 hectare), which is not enough to dilute the downwind plume of toxic drift from the neighbors.

Most of the lots in my neighborhood were empty. There were effectively about three to four acres (about 1.5 hectares) of land per house. This provided more buffering, but barely enough. My neighbor to the south used dryer sheets, which created a plume that reached at least a hundred yards, though it almost always went east of my house. One time her house was spray painted and the wind came directly from the south, so I had to leave immediately and spend the day visiting a friend. A neighbor to the northwest burned firewood all winter, though it was only a problem in February, when the wind came from that direction. On those occasions I sometimes had to sleep with a mask on, and only do laundry on days without smoke.

A more bizarre example of toxic drift happened to someone else in the area. Her neighbor put a large number of mothballs in a circle around the house to keep snakes away. Fortunately using mothballs that way is against the law in Arizona, so it got stopped.

If I moved out beyond the power grid, land became a lot cheaper and houses were further apart. Land well beyond the power grid is slow to be developed with less chance of later surprises. Cell towers are rarely built in such areas, as they need a lot of electricity.

If I moved out there, I could afford four of the lots, so I would have five acres (2 hectares) as a buffer, though I really think ten acres is a much better size.

I had been interested in solar energy for years and was confident I could set up a solar system for lighting and a few other small loads, that all could run on a simple 12 volt system similar to what is used in small RVs.

Fancier solar systems use an inverter to make 110 volt AC electricity from the solar panels, but all types of inverters send out a lot of EMF and dirty electricity, so I did not want one. The only real need I had for 110 volts was to run the washing machine, and I could use a small propane generator for that.

The other appliances, i.e. stove, refrigerator, water heater and boiler, could be run on propane. Propane is a problem for people with MCS, but these appliances would all be in a separate utility shed or outside.

I would have water delivered to a storage tank, rather than drill my own well, which is what most houses in Dolan had.

A critical issue was telephone service. I could not live without a land line, as I could not use a cell phone. I contacted the local phone company, which told me that they would extend a line up to 1000 ft (300 m) for free. Beyond that, it cost $1 per foot, so extending the line for a mile would cost more than $4,000. Fortunately, there were already phone lines out to some remote parts of the Dolan area.

As cell phone usage continues to get cheaper, landline telephone companies are losing customers. I expect rural landlines to eventually become unaffordable and be dismantled in most areas, but I wasn't aware of that issue in those days.

I named this whole idea Remote Basic. It was doable in the Dolan area and climate, and it was possible with the money I had available. It would be very rustic, but it would cover the basic necessities and it would be more comfortable than the porch I was living on and the refugee camp I lived in before. My living expenses would be very low, so I hoped to save enough money to build a real house some years later.

An unusual setup like this would not raise eyebrows in Dolan, but in most other places neighbors might complain to the zoning authorities. This type of setup works best when done discretely, such as in remote areas or on heavily wooded lots. Garden sheds are usually too small to require inspection, though many jurisdictions have a minimum size for dwellings. Zoning enforcement is often relaxed in rural areas and may just respond to neighbor's complaints. I saw no problems doing this in rural Mohave county. Counties with more expensive real estate are usually more strict — including in remote areas without electricity or paved roads.

I know one woman who got in trouble with the zoning in her county after a real estate agent complained. She convinced the board to hold a special hearing on her rural property so they could better understand her situation, but they still refused to grant her a variance.

I know another woman who was forced to sell her remote cabin because of a homeowner's association. Areas covered by such an organization are simply best avoided.

Remote Basic was an enticing idea. I kept thinking about it and refining the details, but I hesitated. Would I get better if I moved? Would I be able to drive again? Could I live remotely if I could not drive? How to find suitable land, when I could not drive around and look? How to manage the construction project? What if, what if.

My current situation was not too bad. I was not uncomfortable sleeping on the porch, I was able to get the groceries I needed and I could hike or bicycle to Dolan. My mind was foggy most of the time, but I had forgotten what a clear mind was like. The days just passed by, one after the other. It was easy to give in to inertia, hope for a miracle and be paralyzed by all the "what ifs."

In the spring of 2005, I heard that a large tract of land three miles south of Meadview was being subdivided. Meadview is about 30 miles (45 km) from Dolan and 40 miles (60 km) from Kingman. Meadview itself had a post office, library, small hardware store and gas station with a convenience store. That wasn't much, but I could reach them on a bicycle.

A friend came up from Tucson to look at the land. A few others were interested, though not right away. We thought of buying up adjacent lots for ourselves and to sell to other people later. We hoped this could be the start of an EI community.

The owner was not really interested in talking to us and he eventually sold the whole tract to a speculator. That was less work for him.

The real estate bubble came to the area at this time, after bidding up nearby Las Vegas to stellar prices. Now speculators discovered the low land prices in the Dolan-Meadview area. Speculators snapped up any land they could find and quickly sold it again to other speculators at inflated prices. People bought land they had never seen, even land that was unbuildable. One speculator knocked on people's doors, asking if they had empty land they would sell.

Someone in Dolan had bought a lot for $5,000 two years before, and now he sold it for $32,000. The asking price for a ten-acre lot near Meadview went as high as $210,000. Even remote lots, very far from paved roads and any utilities, jumped from $2,500 to $16,000 in a short time.

The sudden run-up in land prices put an end to my housing plans in Dolan. The overheated market collapsed a few years later and the land prices came back to normal levels, but I had moved away by then.

I never built Remote Basic. Doing that would probably have been an adventure worth writing a book about, but I'm glad I didn't do it. One problem was that it was too hot for too many months. I used to love a hot day, but later it made me dizzy every afternoon for months at a time.

I since discovered the book *Rancho Costa Nada – The Dirt Cheap Desert Homestead,* by Phil Garlington. He actually lived in such a setup, though his reasons were not health related, and I can't recommend his building methods for anyone with MCS. However, it is a fascinating story of inventiveness and simplicity, and about the interesting characters in his remote corner of the Mojave Desert.

10. The Turnaround

My life in Dolan was coasting along, despite my efforts to improve the situation. Most of the time was really wasted, compared to the productive life I was used to before, but I had made peace with it, so it didn't bother me anymore.

I hiked around the neighborhood a couple of times each day in nearly any kind of weather. In the summer I hiked before sunrise and after sunset, when the heat was manageable. The summer afternoons were too hot to do anything other than have a long siesta, just like the rabbits, birds and other wildlife. Few humans ventured outside their cooled houses during the afternoon heat.

In the winter I often sat in the sun-heated car instead of inside the cold house. Sleeping outside on the porch worked well most of the time. A few times I woke up smelling woodsmoke, but then I put on a mask and went back to sleep. My lungs were irritated by the end of the winter, but it didn't last.

I only slept inside the house a few times when the wind drove rain or snow onto my cot. Then I woke up the next morning with little red bumps on my skin and my lungs felt cold and heavy.

I read several books I never would have had time to read in my previous hectic life as an engineer. I discovered the Arizona author Edward Abbey, whose love of the desert is legendary and his humorous anarchistic distaste for billboards and other commercial ugliness even more so. Another local author I liked was Tony Hillerman and his stories about two Navajo policemen whose intimate knowledge of the tribal religion and culture allow them to solve the mysteries.

I also read some of Elaine Aron's books about Highly Sensitive People, which I found to be very profound.

Reading was complicated as I was very sensitive to both the ink and the paper itself. I had to keep the book inside a cellophane bag and use a pencil with an eraser head to flip the pages. That helped a lot, though it wasn't airtight so I still got dizzy after awhile. Later on, someone gave me a non-electric reading box. It also leaked ink fumes, but it took longer before I got dizzy.

Since I had no radio, TV or computer, my only source of news was the magazine *Newsweek*, which at that time had a different format and was available on paper. The magazine had ads for a new drug called Lyrica, which did a lot for the acceptance of fibromyalgia, as if the illness didn't exist before there was a drug for it. Do we really have to wait for a drug company to make MCS and EHS "acceptable?"

After being stuck for a year, I woke up one cold January morning and was depressed. I could barely get out of bed, as that seemed pointless. It only lasted a few days and has never happened before or since, but it gave me sympathy for people who have to deal with that. It is hard to comprehend what any illness means if we haven't experienced it ourselves.

My situation in Dolan was certainly much better than it had been in the Texas camp, but I was not ready to live like that forever. I was also keenly aware that it was not a stable long-term situation. All sorts of problems could appear and make the present situation unlivable.

One such reminder was a wildfire that burned some square miles of brushland on the side of Mt. Perkins, 15 miles (24 km) to the west. I could see the flames at night and the fire generated a big plume of smoke, but I was fortunately never downwind of it. Without transportation I was a sitting duck.

By the fall of 2005 I had been unable to drive for 18 months. I started to feel burning sensations every afternoon. I did not know the cause of it, but time was clearly not on my side any more. It was time to look at more serious measures.

While I lived in Texas, I was treated by both Dr. William Rea and an alternative health practitioner named Deborah Singleton. Both were more helpful than anybody else I had tried, so it made sense to go back to them, but how to get there? Perhaps I needed a boost.

The first summer I lived in Arizona, I was summoned to Prescott for a reevaluation by my disability insurance company. The physician's office was right next to a power line and any request for accommodations was ignored, so I was forced to be there for 1½ hours. I became seriously overloaded, but fortunately I had an appointment with an alternative health practitioner the next day.

His treatment was similar to what I had experienced in Dallas and he was able to pull me out of the reaction. I went back to him several times, but he was unable to help me further.

Now, two years later, I wondered if he could patch me up enough that I could limp on to Dallas. I thought if I could just drive 200 miles (320 km) a day, I could make it there on my own. He agreed to work on me over three days, if I could come to Sedona.

A friend in Tucson came up and drove me to Verde Valley, where we spent each night at the Dead Horse Ranch state park near Cottonwood. I didn't feel well in the main campground because of the current running in the soil. This is a common problem in campgrounds with electric pedestals at each campsite and can be easily measured with a gaussmeter. Fortunately, the annex campground was wired better and I had no problems there.

The practitioner had borrowed a beautiful underground house for our sessions. It was located in a rural part of Verde Valley, built of natural materials and the electricity was turned off. I felt very good there. He and his wife worked on me each morning until noon.

After three days, I was ready to try driving myself and I drove my car for 45 minutes up and down the interstate. It was definitely better, but I couldn't do it multiple times a day, so I could not continue on to Dallas.

Disappointed, we returned to Dolan and my friend left. At home I noticed that the mysterious burning sensations in the afternoon had become worse. I simply had to get to Dallas. I contacted my friend in Tucson again and asked if he was interested in a long all-expenses paid trip to Dallas.

We left for Dallas two weeks later. It was then the start of October and we were fortunate to have great weather for what turned into a five-week trip.

The first night we camped in a friend's yard east of Tucson. The second night was spent at the City of Rocks State Park in New Mexico, which has an exceptionally good campground for people with MCS and EHS, as it is spread out over a wide area and most sites have no electricity. We talked to a fellow camper who had incurable cancer. She had sold her house and bought a camper van to tour the country while she still could.

The third night we camped in West Texas. The park by Monahan's was full, so we had to camp on the edge of a big oilfield — upwind from the pumps.

It took us four days to make it to Dallas, as I couldn't stand the car for more than a couple of hours at a time, even in the back seat of my very-low-EMF car.

They were all ready for me at Deborah Singleton's clinic. Extra staff had been called in, and they worked on me non-stop for two hours. Their treatments seem similar to what I have read about Therapeutic Touch and some other types of energy work, though I don't really understand how such "energy work" affects the human body. The closest explanation I've seen is the book *Hands of Light* by Barbara Brennan, which leaves a lot of room for the skeptic.

I do not understand how antibiotic pills work either, but I accept that they do work. The physicians know how they work, but if I could travel a hundred years back in time, I doubt many physicians would accept that such a pill was possible.

I did not have the luxury of waiting for scientific clarity but had to go with what seemed to help. And it did help. The mysterious burning sensation that came every afternoon stopped after a few days of treatment, even though I still had no idea what caused it. This was very encouraging.

This type of treatment obviously requires a skill that is not easily obtained. In Arizona I tried three such practitioners — only one of them seemed to have any positive effect, and it was not enough.

We settled into a routine visiting Dr Rea's clinic in the morning, Deborah Singleton's in the afternoon and returning to our campground on the north shore of Lake Lewisville, near the town of Hickory Creek.

The campground was owned by the U.S. Army Corps of Engineers and sat on a peninsula sticking out into the lake, so the air quality was very good. We mostly stayed at one campsite where I put my tent on a tiny wooded peninsula, so I would get the breeze from the lake and rarely any woodsmoke. My friend slept in the car.

The bathhouses had two-story cathedral ceilings and no fragrances. They were so safe that my friend slept on a bench in there for a few nights after the car got contaminated by a leaking fuel line.

Campgrounds are often difficult during weekends, with a clientele that tends to have smoky campfires, barbecues and noisy parties. We avoided that by spending two weekends at a friend's house in the country, two hours' drive east of Dallas.

I was ready to go home after more than three weeks of daily treatments. I felt better and tried to drive the car myself while we were in New Mexico; it was better, but not great. I was taught various yoga-like exercises, which should help me get better over time, so I still had hope.

We visited the EI community in Rodeo, New Mexico on the way back. We stayed for a week while camping in various people's yards, on public land and even one night at a playground. At the playground we hung around until dark before setting up the tent, so nobody got suspicious. The next morning two men from Mexico walked by and asked for food and water. The border was only 30 miles (50 km) away, so there was a lot of such traffic.

One of the couples there were building their own house. They did not have a bank loan so they camped on their land and used the saved "rent" to buy materials a little at a time. They lived in an old renovated Airstream travel trailer, but he was too sensitive to sleep inside with his wife and had to sleep in an old car. It took them seven years, but it became a beautiful and safe house. It was built with walls of rock and mortar, with a steel roof and a floor of bricks set in sand.

I considered moving to Rodeo and looked for vacant land, which mostly consisted of 40-acre (16 hectare) lots. The real estate "bubble" had just arrived, with speculators buying up land for whatever the sellers were asking. The prices went up almost daily; lots that were affordable six months earlier were now out of reach. The only parcel the realtor could offer in my price range was located on the appropriately named Stuck Truck Road (it has since been renamed). Both the lot and the road became a muddy hell during the two-month monsoon every summer.

I tried looking for a private deal instead. One of the EI families suggested we try to split a 40-acre parcel sandwiched between their ranch and a large tract of public land. That might bring the cost into my price range. The owner wasn't sure she would sell or not and eventually we gave up.

Rodeo was very isolated. The nearest stores with organic foods and building materials were in Silver City and Bisbee, which both were 70 to 80 miles (110 to 130 km) away. It would have been difficult to move there without my own transportation.

We returned to Dolan in the middle of November. The weather then got much colder and I had to close up the house for the winter. I always felt worse in the winter and this was no exception.

I didn't try to drive my car all winter; I wanted to wait until I felt better in the spring, so there was a better chance for success. I didn't need a spectacular failure to destroy my confidence.

I felt better when spring arrived and I could spend more time outside. I had done the daily yoga-like exercises they taught me in Dallas and that seemed helpful as well.

I started cautiously experimenting with the car on very short trips, where I made sure not to overdo it. I paid close attention and noticed that it seemed to work better if I first walked around the neighborhood for an hour right before driving, so I made sure to repeat that.

I could drive to Dolan, rest for ten minutes while doing some of the yoga exercises, then drive home again.

Some days later I did the walk-around, drove to Dolan, rested, then drove to visit a nearby friend and then home.

I gradually expanded the routine, while staying in the immediate area so I never overdid it. It seemed optimal if the first driving segment was 10 minutes long. As I added more segments, I seemed to sense the car less. Perhaps my body adjusted to it — or it just got numbed.

Eventually, I drove the thirty miles (50 km) to the town of Meadview, with a few rest stops on the way. I had a friend there, who could help me home if needed, but it worked fine. I was elated that I was able to get that far on my own.

It was a grand feeling when I soon after arrived in Kingman under my own steam. I then started doing my own shopping in Kingman. Things were really looking up, and I could live with the rest stops it took to get there. One of the other people in Dolan had been doing a similar procedure for some time, though sometimes she fell asleep during her rest stops.

Eventually I got even bolder. On a particularly good day, I drove to Kingman, hopped on Interstate 40 and headed east. I turned around at a truck stop twenty miles out of town and headed back, passed Kingman and out to Yucca west of Kingman, then back to Kingman and home to Dolan. I had travelled 150 miles (240 km) in 20-minute segments. It had taken all day, but it worked. The next day I drove to Kingman and back again, just to make sure there was no major fallout — there wasn't.

Like the Apollo space program, I had gradually gotten further and further away from home, while learning how much I could handle. Now it was time to see if I could do what had seemed like a moon-shot just two months earlier.

11. *Crossing the Void*

I had a pen friend who lived in an EI community in the high desert of northeastern Arizona, near a town with the curious name Snowflake. We had talked about arranging transport so I could visit and look for better housing there, but now it looked like I might drive there myself.

I looked at the map: it was 320 miles (510 km) from Dolan Springs, with most of it by freeway. I had proven that I could drive 150 miles in one day, so I should be able to do the trip in two long days. It was mid-June 2006, time to make a bold move.

I left sooner than expected, as a wildfire started twenty miles southwest of Dolan, with smoke drifting our way. Just two days after my proof-of-concept drive up and down Interstate 40, I packed up my car with food, water, camping gear and whatever else I would need for a lengthy trip. I expected to be gone a week or two, but it became more than four weeks.

The trip started out like the regular trips to Kingman. I drove for about twenty minutes, then rested until any symptoms were gone. I passed Kingman and headed east on Interstate 40. It went well.

Then there was a long stretch of freeway without exits. I could feel I was overdoing it, and was relieved when I finally came to exit 109. It was lunchtime and I rested for an hour under a big juniper bush.

The rest did not restore me, and I could feel the car soon after taking off. Okay, I'd dealt with that before and just driven shorter sections. But there was longer between the freeway exits than I would have liked, and there was no forest to camp in before I got to Ash Fork.

I pressed on, made it to Ash Fork and went south on highway 89. After seven miles, I found an unmarked Forest Service road, drove in and soon found a place to camp for the night. It was just a spot with no facilities of any kind, but there were no people or any other problems. It was free and legal, and I had done such rustic camping many times before.

I woke up the next morning with an "EMF hangover," which to me feels like a tingling sensation. When I tried to sit in my car, I got stronger symptoms, even though the car was modified to be absolutely EMF-free without the ignition on.

I have had this experience before. After an overexposure I am even more sensitive than usual and it seems that all the metal in the car is then affecting me. How that can be is a mystery that I hope some open-minded scientist will figure out some day.

I was clearly not able to sit in the car, let alone turn on the engine and drive it. I had plenty of food and water, so it was no problem to stay put and wait it out. I was not really worried.

I hiked along the Forest Service road in the cool morning and evening, while the heat of the day was spent in the shade of a big juniper bush. I didn't see a single person all day.

The next morning, I felt better, though I had not fully recovered. I knew there were various places to camp for the next sixty miles (95 km), so I could do the rest of the trip over two days if needed. The freeway exits were also closer together for the rest of the trip.

I drove cautiously, with shorter sections on the road, and longer rest periods. That seemed to work. Soon I was walking around the town of Williams, while gawking at the Route 66 nostalgia.

When I came to the end of Kaibab National Forest, east of Flagstaff, I knew there were no more places to camp. I either had to stop there for the night or commit to going all the way to Snowflake that day — I continued.

There was major road construction in Winslow that kept me in the car for too long. I was wearing out, but still making it.

At a deserted exit past Winslow, I was asked for help by another motorist who had run out of fuel. I felt bad about it, but I didn't have it in me to drive him back to Winslow to get some fuel. Having a "normie" and a fuel canister in my car would also be a hazard, even on a good day.

I reached my destination late in the day, much to my relief. My pen friend and two of her neighbors gave me a warm welcome.

My pen friend was not able to offer lodging herself, but someone else had offered that I could camp in her yard. It was common for visitors to the community to camp there.

I was burned out on driving for several days, but my pen friend drove me around the area in the back seat of her low-EMF diesel car.

I didn't really have any plans beyond making it to Snowflake, but I found it a fascinating place. There were eight EI houses in a little neighborhood out in the country (by 2019 the cluster had grown to fourteen houses). Each house was on a 20 acre (8 hectare) or larger lot, as required by the zoning. Additional houses were scattered over a larger area.

Three new houses were under construction, and there were plans for even more. The state of Arizona was also planning to build four rental houses for people with environmental illness, who were on a low income. People talked about construction all the time; it was like a fever in the air.

Almost everyone who lived there at the time had built their own homes. As modern-day pioneers, they had left their home states and travelled to Arizona with the hope of a better life, and they often had to live under primitive conditions while their houses were built. This meant that the people living there had a much more positive "can-do" spirit than I had seen any other place. I found that very appealing.

I learned that the first MCS house in the community was finished in 1988, by an engineer who had to flee the polluted air in the Phoenix metro area. Back in those days most of the MCS houses were not successful, but his was. In the following years, more people moved to the area and built homes, while slowly developing the methods for building MCS houses. Today, almost all the houses built using these methods are successful, largely thanks to the pioneering efforts of one resident: Bruce McCreary.

I have visited so many MCS houses that I did not feel good in, including many of the houses in Dolan Springs, but here in Snowflake I felt fine in most of them. I even did pretty well in one that was not even fully completed; the walls were closed in and sealed, but the floor was still raw concrete. A couple of months later, I visited the same house again. The floor was now tiled and the walls had been painted a week before with clay paint. I felt fine. I was very impressed. Here was a place that had proven knowledge of how to build safe houses, and contractors experienced in doing it.

I had expected to stay for about a week, but I was so intrigued that I kept hanging around. Then I was invited to a great Independence Day party for the whole EI community. It was held outdoors, with lots of great food. Some of the dishes even had little labels with the ingredients to help those with food allergies.

About twenty people attended the party, including two other people who were looking for a better place to live — just like myself. One of them was a woman from Tucson with a small RV, which she later moved to Dolan Springs, to camp in my yard while looking around that area.

Later that summer, a guy from Georgia came through, and one day a car with Idaho plates came up the driveway. She had been living in her car for a while and one day she asked a gas station attendant to fill up her car, explaining that if she did it herself, the fumes would make her sick. The attendant then told her that his father (or uncle) lived in a little town down in Arizona where there were lots of people with this problem. She thought she was the only one in the world with this illness. Intrigued, she headed down to Arizona. When she came to Snowflake, she went into the grocery store and asked where she could find people like herself. Someone gave her directions to the EI neighborhood. She first knocked on someone's door, who then directed her to the house where I was staying, which is where most visitors ended up in those days.

Every year, several people drive around the Southwest looking for safe housing. Most sleep in their car, some bring tents or a travel trailer. Some find a place to stay, some go home empty-handed. A few continue to camp around the state. The campgrounds around Tucson have served as a winter haven for many homeless people with EI over the years.

The documentary movie *Homesick – Living with Multiple Chemical Sensitivities,* tells the story of Susan Abod's journey to the Southwest in search of safe housing. She converted a van to live in, which gave her much more comfortable accommodations than most people have on such a trip. She travelled around Texas, Arizona and New Mexico and eventually settled in Santa Fe.

The town of Snowflake looked much nicer than most desert towns, with its trees and gardens around old brick homes. It had most of the stores I needed, with more available in the surrounding towns.

There were small, irrigated farms around town, while further out it was all ranchland. A bumper sticker sums it up nicely: *Eat beef – the West wasn't won on salad.*

The mile-high (1600 meter) elevation created a much milder summer than the brutal heat in the low desert. I felt good there. I had not yet experienced the cold winters and the bone-rattling winds in the spring, but they are not so bad with a well-built house.

After visiting for two weeks, it was clear that my future was here.

12. *Finding the Land*

Once I decided to look for land, I was told that a 20 acre (8 hectare) lot was for sale close to the EI neighborhood. It was a great lot at a price I could afford. I had never bought real estate before and was learning how that worked. The owner told me that we could work directly with a title company and save the ten percent a realtor would charge.

It seemed like the perfect deal, but there was one problem: every time I visited the land, I felt a tingling sensation and stiffness in my joints, as if I was exposed to electromagnetic fields. This was very puzzling, as there were no nearby houses, power lines or cell towers and the instruments I had showed very little radiation.

The owner gave me permission to camp on his land, so I could better check it out. I drove over there one afternoon, left the car where the dirt road ended, carried my camping gear to the middle of the lot and set up the tent. I had a terrible night; I woke up feeling like the ground was vibrating. It wasn't, but one of the symptoms I can get from EMF exposures somehow makes my nervous system act that way.

I normally sleep soundly every night, except when I get exposed to chemicals or EMF. If I get exposed during the day, the symptoms can sometimes show up later. What could have caused this? Perhaps that I drove there? Then why did that not happen where I normally camped? I tried camping there a second night with the same result.

I remembered that when I lived in Texas some heavy thunderstorms could produce these symptoms in me. I didn't have any problems with the thunderstorms in Dolan, but there were more of them here. But they didn't disturb me when I camped in my regular place, so that wasn't it, either.

I camped several times on the land, but it never worked and it was wearing me down, so I started to have these symptoms every afternoon no matter where I was. The woman in whose yard I was camping asked me to walk with her to a big open area with no houses. After being there in the bright sun for awhile, she asked if I was feeling any better. I wasn't.

She told me that a lot of us are sensitive to light and that could be my problem. We walked back to her house, which had small windows that were partially covered with aluminum sheets. She brought out more sheets and a roll of aluminum tape and fully covered all the windows. She then invited me to stay inside her darkened house for a couple of days.

For the next two days I stayed inside the house from sunrise to sunset. After sunset I went for a walk before I set up the tent for the night.

I felt a lot better doing that. When I ventured out in the sunshine on the third day it was clear that I was sensitive to sunlight. It was the cause of various mysterious symptoms I'd had for the last couple of years, including those afternoon burning sensations that had forced me to travel to Dallas the year before. The tinglings I sometimes felt at sunrise were also the light sensitivity.

Since I was outside all day, this photosensitivity had gotten worse on the trip, and since it came on slowly, I had not been able to make the connection. This was a great "aha" moment.

Someone else came over and showed me some special sun protection clothes and extra-dark sunglasses she used. I express-ordered a set from Sun Precautions and NoIR Medical. The clothes and the glasses were easy to clean up so they did not smell and really helped me with the light sensitivity.

Sensitivity to sunlight is common in the EI world. I knew one person in Dolan avoided sunlight and now I learned there were also people like that in Snowflake. It is not just a problem for people living in the sunny desert. I have since heard of people with that problem living in darker places, such as Seattle, England and Finland. I have read about people with such severe light sensitivity they had to live in almost total darkness, including authors Diana Crumpler and Anna Lyndsey, as well as Hannelore Kohl, the First Lady of Germany.

I had to hurry home to Dolan to keep an important appointment, but before I left, I told the landowner that he could go ahead with the title company.

I drove back to Dolan in two days, camping one night at the same place south of Ash Fork. I felt better in the car, though I still needed to stop for a rest every twenty minutes.

Three weeks later I was back in Snowflake, with about a week left before we closed on the land deal. I went over to visit the land that was soon to be mine, and was very surprised that I still felt bad over there. I had not visited the land since the discovery that I was photosensitive, and had just assumed that was the whole problem. It was not. There was something else . . . but what?

I went camping over there for a couple of nights, and I again woke up feeling as if my body was vibrating. On the second night I had to walk around for an hour around midnight to be able to sleep. I never have to do that.

Someone suggested I ask a dowser, and I was told about two in the area. I asked both of them to come. They came on separate days and they essentially told me the same thing:

that they could detect "something," but they could not explain what it was.

They both said the western edge of the land was better so I tried to camp there for a night and did well. But I didn't want my house built there — there were a lot of junipers and it was close to the lot line. I was concerned that a house could later be built close-by on the adjacent lot (which happened three years later).

It also didn't seem wise to build a house that close to this mysterious problem.

I seemed to feel fine on both the western and eastern edges of the land and if I walked well into the adjacent lots to the north and south. This meant the problem couldn't be anything outside the lot, it had to be something on the lot, but there wasn't anything other than the usual bare desert. I was not sure what to make of this. The closing date was coming up very soon, so I had to make a decision. I decided to make one last full-scale test.

My friend blocked her windows again, and I sat in her house until well after sunset. Then I hiked over to the land in the darkness, and started feeling the tingling once I got there. I hiked ½ mile back and sat down — no tingling. I hiked back to the land, and started to tingle. I hiked ½ mile away again, and again there was no tingling.

I cancelled the purchase. I don't know what the problem was, but I could not live there. Anyone with a scientific education would be very skeptical of an investigation relying on a single human test subject. Humans are not reliable "instruments." It is only because I was able to repeat the problem so many times, while eliminating any other explanation, that I believed it myself. I've been told that it might be "geopathic stress," though I don't really understand what that is.

After this was all over, two other people told me that they also had trouble being over there. One of them wanted to buy the lot a year earlier and also gave up. I visited the land four years later and it was no better then.

I was very disappointed. The lot seemed so perfect and I could afford it. The real-estate bubble had reached Snowflake and people were starting to demand sky-high prices in the hope some speculator would pay it. A 20-acre lot in the same neighborhood went on the market with an asking price of $73,000 — nearly three times recent prices. It looked like a repeat of what happened six months earlier in Rodeo and a year before in the Dolan area.

I brooded over this misfortune for a few days. Then a friend resolutely said we should go see a realtor she knew. The realtor gave us directions to various lots in the area and we spent the day driving around to look at them. None of it was suitable, but it got me rolling again.

I decided I really needed to look around with an open mind — to cast a wide net and see what came up. I started to roam over a wide area and drove down several dirt roads to see what was there. I was surprised to see houses in all sorts of remote areas, even several miles down dirt roads.

At the foot of a big mesa I discovered a secluded valley that looked promising. I talked to some of the people living there and they told me most houses were heated with firewood and the low areas were often filled with the blue haze of smoke during the winter. They also told me there was no cell phone reception and they all looked forward to a tower that was planned for the mesa next door (it was built eight years later).

I looked at areas further away and discovered some remote subdivisions around Concho and along highway 180 and Interstate 40. These subdivisions were largely empty, with just a few scattered houses. The lots were affordable, but they were too far away from the EI neighborhood for me to have a social life.

I visited a 40-acre lot that was about twenty miles (32 km) east of Holbrook, near the main entrance to the Petrified Forest National Park. The only house in the entire subdivision was on the adjacent lot. The owner saw me walking around and came out to talk to me. He told me he could not find a contractor willing to commute to his building site, so he hired a man who lived on the land in a trailer while building the house. When the house was finished, the contractor moved on to the next job. That worked out well, but it was still difficult to get a handyman to come out from Holbrook to make repairs.

The lot was about a mile from the freeway. A few years later, there were no less than three cell phone towers erected nearby.

Then one day I decided to try something different. I drove to the end of a dirt road that ran only a few miles from the EI neighborhood. I left my car where the road ended and hiked down a jeep trail. A mile along this path, the trail ended at a house on top of a small hill where I could see for miles in all directions. I could see a house on another hill that I recognized as one I'd seen before from a dirt road coming in from the other side.

It was a very sparsely populated area, with little vegetation and miles away from any towers and electrical service. It seemed so remote, even though it was only five miles (8 km) from the nearest paved road. Without grid power, development is slow, land prices low and the chance of a cell tower very small.

I had pretty much decided my house should be powered by the sun anyway, so it was not a problem that there was no electrical service. I actually considered it a plus.

I now totally focused on this area, which was remote enough that it was passed over by the speculators. If I hired a road grader to upgrade and extend the jeep trail for another mile, then my drive to Snowflake and the EI neighborhood would be 12 miles (19 km) shorter than the existing road.

There was an empty house with a "For Sale" sign on it. It had a garage built of concrete blocks, that I might be able to live in if I fixed it up with insulation and drywall on the inside. The main house was a wooden structure in poor condition. It had forty fenced-in acres and a well with a windmill pumper. The owner wanted $90,000. I would need to spend a lot of money to fix up the place, so the total cost would be the same if I built a house myself, and the result would be much better.

The County administration was very helpful, providing me maps showing how the area was divided into lots in sizes from 20 acres and up to a few thousand acres, so I knew what I was looking at. It was just open land with no fences or much else to give an idea how it was subdivided.

I roamed around the area and looked at everything. A friend drove me around the area one afternoon in her pickup truck where we went down some jeep trails my car could not make it through. One of these trails ended abruptly with a sheer drop of about 15 feet (5 meters), without any warning. Some parts had no trails at all, so I hiked in there on foot to look around.

I camped three nights in separate parts of the area to see how I felt. I felt wonderful there. I loved it so far from everything. Camping there also taught me some important things. The first place I camped, the ground was solid rock just below a thin layer of sand, so I could not even get a tent peg in. I asked a contractor about how to build a septic system in such a place, and he said I could build an above-ground system, but it was expensive and needed a lot of electricity for the pumps.

Most lots were too big, one had a lot of junk on it and I wanted a lot with no road frontage, to avoid the road dust.

There were no sale signs on any of the lots, but I decided to send a letter to some owners and see if they were interested. I selected six lots and the county office in Holbrook gave me the owners' mailing addresses. One owner responded — he owned the lot I liked the best.

He said he bought the lot twenty years ago with the intent of retiring there. His wife had just died and he realized he was comfortable where he was, and he was about to call a realtor when my letter arrived. He said he wanted a no-hassle deal, no dickering around, his price was final. Then he stated his price: it was about half what I had expected. I nearly fell off the chair.

My first attempt at buying land taught me how to work with a title agency, which is quite easy. No need for any realtor or attorney. I rushed in to the title agency and told them I wanted to pay all fees, even those customarily paid by the seller. I wanted it done as smooth and fast as possible and not give the seller any excuse to reconsider the sale or the price. The fees totaled $550.

The agency had to do a title search and get the seller's notarized signature. Meanwhile, I hired a service to do the percolation test for the septic system and spent a lot of time on the land to decide where the house should be and find the little survey markers in the corners, which was not easy.

The percolation test was done on a cold October morning. A backhoe dug holes to get soil samples, which were tested for how fast water moved through them. This ensured that my future sewage system could work properly. I could not get a building permit without this test. If the test failed, I would not buy the land, but it passed fine and the inspector then specified the size of the septic leach field based on the test. I drove home to Dolan two days later. The sale closed ten days later. The land was now mine.

13. Planning the House

The winter in Dolan Springs was spent planning my new house. I had thought about housing on and off for years, but it is different once it is for real.

I wanted to make sure the house was well built, as repairs and maintenance can be very disruptive for someone with MCS, and I wanted it to be warm and comfortable after spending so many winters in a cold house.

It was a great boon that I could follow the proven "Snowflake method." I knew from first-hand experience that this method worked for me. It was a lot easier to plan the house when I could use the same basic materials and methods. I still had many choices to make, especially since my house was far from the electrical grid, which was pioneering territory for an EI house.

One woman agreed to be my adviser. I had briefly met her during my 2002 scouting trip to Arizona and again when she came to Dolan Springs to look at three EI houses that were for sale at that time. She wasn't able to spend a night in any of the three houses – nobody could at the time, that's why they were for sale. Instead she slept in mine during her visit. She then moved into an apartment in the EI neighborhood in Snowflake and a couple of years later she started building a house there. Her house was nearly finished when I bought my land. I felt fine inside her house, even though it wasn't quite finished yet. Hers was a success to follow. It was very helpful to walk into her house and see how a certain detail was done, and to have someone to ask things like whether we should tile the floors before sealing the walls (answer: no) and how many inches there should be between the commode and the wall. During the construction she gave me advance information about the next steps, so I could be prepared for them.

This was all tremendously helpful. Some people have a problem following other people's advice; their ego gets in the way, and they have to do it their own way. Sometimes that works, but I've seen several cases where they ran into serious trouble that could easily have been avoided.

There seemed to be no shortage of advice offered by other people. Some was offered with great confidence, even by people who had never built a house themselves, or by those who built a house they could not live in. I stuck to the advice of two people: my adviser, and occasionally the guy who had mentored her.

A Home Depot building supply store had just opened in Kingman. Since there was also a Home Depot within forty miles (60 km) of my land in Snowflake, I could check out some materials in advance. The problem was that even with my respirator on, I could be inside for only fifteen minutes before I got dizzy. I once used up that time standing in line at the pro desk. When I realized that was not gonna work, I asked the clerk if he could look up the information and then I would come back in again ten minutes later to retrieve it. When I came back in, the clerk had done nothing and just told me there were other people in line. Obviously, I had to stand there to hold my place in line — he could not just think of me in the line and do the task when it was my turn. It was the height of a building boom, so they were busy and there was no sympathy for my special need.

A great variety of filter cartridges were available for my 3M 6200 respirator. Perhaps something else could work better than the "VOC" filter I was using. I tried various kinds and found the "Multi Gas/Vapor" cartridge worked better. I could now be inside Home Depot for an hour.

I visited the county planning and zoning department before I left Snowflake. They gave me some materials about their building requirements, which was basically that the International Residential Code must be followed, with some additional local stipulations. In their rack of informational brochures, I found instructions on how to build a code-approved outhouse!

I ordered a copy of the International Residential Code, which is a phone-book sized tome I read over the winter. It was well written and was helpful for some details of the house, such as sizing the vents and sewage pipes, that had to be specified on the plans I submitted for approval.

I also read a general book about home construction (*Do-It-Yourself Housebuilding* by George Nash), which was very helpful in giving me an idea of the whole process and some of the new words I needed to learn. There is a lot to learn to build a successful house, even though the details may seem overwhelming.

I had to call a few vendors, but it was really hard to get to talk to a human. Even sales departments did not return phone calls if they knew I was not from some corporation. One time I complained to a phone operator, who indignantly responded that of course they would call me back — and of course they didn't. One vendor told me they were not sure what price they should charge me, as I was not a contractor.

Sometimes I was simply referred to a website and when I tried to explain that I could not use a computer I was told to "just go to the library" or "learn to use one." I once tried to say that I actually had a Master's degree in computer engineering and explain the situation — I might as well have said I just landed with a space ship from Mars.

I tried asking questions by postal mail. I received one helpful reply and one that simply stated: "Our website address is . . ."

The various county offices I contacted were no better to answer or call back. Just keep trying.

I needed to get some information from the web, but how to do that without computer access? Someone suggested I hire a lady I had never met. I sent her a letter with what I needed information about, and then heard nothing for weeks. Finally, I sent her a note to stop any further work and send me what she had. She replied that she wanted to finish the work. After several more weeks I got a couple sheets with what she had found and a bill for nine hours of work. I could easily have done this myself in an hour or two, if I could tolerate a computer. I later found someone who was much more proficient and timely.

The lot I bought was forty acres (17 hectares) large with several choices where to place the house. There was a hill on the west end of the land, which many people would consider the obvious building site, but I didn't. I knew that was a very windy location. The hill also shielded my house from a cell tower eight miles further west — a cell phone worked well on top of the hill, but not in the radio-shadow east of the hill.

I also wanted to avoid any low spots, both in case we had torrential rain and also because low spots are colder on calm winter nights.

I wanted to site the house somewhat in the middle, so I had some distance to all the lot lines, in case someone later developed the adjacent empty lots. I knew one guy who put his house at the extreme end of his large lot, and then someone built a house right across the street a few years later. Empty lots do not stay empty forever.

Another consideration was there had to be a place for the septic system that was lower than the house and not too rocky.

I made the decision on where to place the house while I was still in Snowflake, as that was necessary for the percolation test.

I could only afford a small house of about 800 sq. ft (80 m²). I therefore had to use the space efficiently. It is easy to stink up the airspace in a small room with things that are not a problem in a larger room, and an open floor plan also makes a small house seem larger, so I designed the house with as few walls as possible and with no corridor or vestibule. There was just a bathroom, a bedroom and a large L-shaped living room and kitchen.

Cooking odors bothered me, especially if I burned the food, so I had cooked outside all the years in Dolan. I first used an electric hot plate and later a propane camping stove. I planned on continuing that in my new house, otherwise I would need the kitchen to be a separate room to keep the odors out of the rest of the house and I doubted it would work with propane anyway.

If I could afford a larger house, I would add a large walk-in closet or a second bedroom to store my clothes and other things, and then have nothing stored in my bedroom.

The ceiling and all the walls in the bathroom were tiled to protect against mold. This also made it the least smelly room in the house. I designed it so a cot could fit in there in case I needed to sleep there. (I slept there only one single night, but it can be my safe space in case we need to do major repairs on the house someday.)

I put a lot of thought into designing a house that was efficient, supportive of my needs, and adapted to the local climate. These are not priorities for many architects and developers and few houses are built that way.

Some books and articles recommend living on the land for a year before building the house. This is good advice, but not always practical.

If people move to Arizona from another climate, they may bring along ideas of what a house should look like from their old climate, and want the same here. The result may be a house that is great for the cool and cloudy climate of New England, but not for the relentless sun and heat of the desert. The fix is then to put in a large air conditioner and pay a high electrical bill.

One of the Snowflake houses was designed by an architect from another area who was not so familiar with the local climate. The porch and entrance door were placed on the windy side of the house making the porch a lot less usable and the door difficult to handle when the wind blows. The screen door was once pulled right off the hinges by the wind. The house also had big windows on the west side, so the afternoon sun overheated the house.

I learned a lot from the many houses I visited in Snowflake. It was clear that a porch was an important part of an MCS house, to have visitors, open mailed packages, offgas things and much else. It was also clear that my porch should be on the east side, to be out of the wind. The entrance door should also be on the east side, with the north side the acceptable alternative.

The nearby Navajo tribe's religion also specifies the entrance door to be on the east side, traditionally to greet the rising sun every morning.

I also learned that a house needs cross-ventilation that is protected from rain. This is typically a window on each side of the house, protected by a porch roof or some other overhang. There are also special awning windows, which are hinged on the top to provide their own protection from rain.

The windows must be left open as much as possible in a new house to let it offgas. Later on, it is helpful to leave windows open for ventilation on summer nights. Some of the Snowflake houses use a clay paint which is marred if rain comes in through the window and trickles down the wall. I've seen it happen.

I watched one person in Snowflake rush home to close the windows of her new house every time a dark cloud was approaching, which was daily during the monsoon season. It is better not to have to do that.

It was winter in Dolan Springs while I was planning my new house. That was my seventh winter with little or no heat, first in Texas and now in Arizona. I knew the Snowflake winters were colder than those in Dolan and Seagoville and I promised myself that I would never again be cold in my home.

I got through the cold winters in Seagoville by filling up the bathtub with water as hot as I could stand it and then staying in the tub as long as possible. I did the same on the coldest mornings in Dolan. The bathtubs in both places were not deep enough to cover me with water, so I looked into deeper bathtubs. There was a specialty store in Las Vegas, but it turned out to be an upscale luxury boutique, for a clientele far above my finances. I didn't learn anything about bathtubs, but it was interesting to gawk at their $18,000 marble sink and the wealthy clientele.

I did put in a deeper bathtub in my new home, but it was never needed to keep me warm in the winter.

All the MCS houses in Snowflake were at that time heated with electricity. Since my new house would be off the grid, my choice of a heat source was either coal, firewood or propane. Heating the house by the sun alone did not seem practical in the Snowflake winter.

Propane was the easy choice, I just had to put the heater in a sealed closet on the side of the house, so no combustion fumes or leaking gas could get into the house.

A forced-air system was out of the question. Those systems generally have problems with dust, noise, mold and unpleasantly moving air. Propane models also contribute to poor air quality in the house. Some models claim to have sealed combustion chambers, but they still have hot metal in contact with the air and I was very skeptical. My doctor said he'd never seen a safe gas heater.

The only viable heating system was a propane water boiler feeding a hydronic (i.e. water-based) heating system. Such systems use either wall-mounted radiators or an in-floor heating coil. I had never experienced a radiant floor heating system before, while I was familiar with the radiators, so I looked into both.

One reason I chose radiant-floor heating was that it works with a lower water temperature. I was simply not able to find a real water boiler that did not require 110 volt AC electricity for its controls. With floor heating, I could use a simple non-electric propane water heater. These can probably not be used with wall-mounted radiators, as they cannot produce water that is hot enough.

Now I live with radiant floor heating, I know it is far superior to anything else. The only downside is the extra cost, as it requires a more expensive insulated foundation, which will be described later.

I designed the house to also use passive solar heating. This is a method where the building catches the winter sun to help with the heating. It basically means that the windows on the south side are larger, so the winter sun comes in and heats up the tiled floor. A roof overhang blocks the summer sun, when it is higher in the sky and the heat is not wanted.

It is pretty simple, costs very little and has no electronic or mechanical parts. The main hazard is if too many windows are put in the south façade, so the house overheats on winter days and loses too much heat on winter nights.

I designed the house with the living room all along the south wall, so it is well heated by the winter sun, and the warm air then naturally flows into the other parts of the house. I also designed so I had daylight available everywhere and no need for electric lights during the day. Good daylighting is also a mold deterrent. However, I was careful to keep the windows rather small on the west, north and east sides to prevent afternoon overheating in the summer and great heat loss in the winter.

I needed an outbuilding for things I did not want in the house, such as the washing machine, the pumps, the batteries for the solar system, books and items I was offgassing.

I considered using the outbuilding as a temporary home, so I could end the lease in Dolan much sooner. I knew two people who had done that, but they did it while waiting for their new houses to offgas, which can easily take a year if there is exposed drywall and other things to offgas. I fully expected my house to be livable within a few months of completion, so I really just needed temporary lodging for one winter, before the house was finished. That meant I had no heat and no bathroom available, unless I spent a lot of money installing that in the outbuilding.

I could not use an electric space heater, which some people have used in their temporary housing.

If I were building in a milder climate, such as Dolan, I might have done it without any heat, and with a composting or sawdust toilet in a garden shed, but that was not possible with the Snowflake winter.

I considered constructing the outbuilding first, since it was a smaller project and it then could offgas first, just in case. I had plans for a larger outbuilding (I think it was 12 x 20 ft for awhile) with a tiny bathroom for guests camping in my yard, but I postponed that until the main house was finished. That was the right choice, since when the house was finished, I could only scrape money together for a much smaller outbuilding, with no bathroom.

The house was designed to have the basic features other people would want in case I had to sell it. This includes space and hookups for stove, refrigerator, washer and dryer inside the house.

14. Choosing the Materials

A crucial part of planning a healthy house is selecting the building materials. There is no standard set of "safe" materials, as people have different sensitivities. The bibliography section at the end of this book lists other publications about healthy housing. They provide other perspectives and methods that may be more suitable, though be aware that some books (and web sites) assume a lower level of sensitivity than mine, or they assume there is "only" a sensitivity to chemicals or to electromagnetic fields. It is important to know what the issues are and how "safe" a house needs to be.

Several years ago I saw a description of a "healthy house" built by a large, well known non-profit organization. It had carpeting, a fireplace and other features I could not live with, but the house was still healthier than a typical home.

While most people with MCS agree that particle boards and plywood should not be used inside a house, some have no problem with real wood, which others abhor. It takes time to make good choices, and most materials must be chosen before starting on a house.

I had a tremendous advantage since I felt fine inside my adviser's newly built house, so I knew the materials she used also worked for me. That made the choices easier, though I still had some decisions to make.

Manufacturers change the content of their products over time, whether it is caulk, paint, thinset, drywall or other manufactured products. I know some of the products have changed since I selected the materials in 2007, so it does not make sense to list what were my favorite brands at the time. People who are building or renovating today need to do their own testing.

When researching materials, it can be helpful to look up the Material Safety Data Sheet (MSDS) for a product. This information is publicly available to allow firefighters and people transporting or working with a material to check how dangerous it is. Unfortunately, the manufacturers do not have to disclose ingredients that comprise less than 1% of the material (unless it's a recognized carcinogen) and even such small amounts can easily make a product unusable in a healthy house. There are other loopholes in the law that allow manufacturers to hide ingredients that are more than 1% of the material.

Before I visited Snowflake, it was my plan to build all the walls of autoclaved aerated concrete. With a proper coating, these blocks can eliminate the need for siding, insulation, studs and drywall. I tolerated the material very well and there was a factory in Arizona (since closed), so transport costs should be reasonable. There were no contractors available within two hundred miles who had experience building with this material, though I could have paid a local contractor to go to a class in Phoenix.

With no experienced contractor, how could we estimate the cost of the house? Would it cost more than the alternative method? There were other issues, such as how to safely and economically super-insulate such a house. And with no local experience, what surprises would we run into? It was tempting to try this material, but it was less risky to do what I had seen work so well.

We used steel barn siding for the walls with wooden studs, fiberglass insulation and sealed gypsum drywall. This will be described in detail in a later chapter. A great benefit of building with steel is that it is generally less odorous than many other materials, it is very durable, requires no paint for several decades, and is cheaper to use than most other less-toxic materials. The steel siding also provides shielding against cell towers and other microwave transmitters if I need it in the future. This is discussed in the chapter about shielding.

We used a lot of aluminum foil to seal the walls. That is a low-cost material that is well-tolerated by most. The foil is dull on one side and shiny on the other. Someone insisted this was because there was a plastic coating on one side and I should be careful how I mounted the foil. I doubted that was true, since foils are used for cooking, but to make sure I wrote a letter to a large manufacturer. I simply asked if there was a coating on it and if it should be on the outside or inside when used to wrap food on a grill. I did not mention any health concerns. The company obviously received this question a lot. They responded with a form letter explaining in some detail how their manufacturing process leaves the foil shiny on one side and matte on the other. There was no coating. A "non-stick" foil product with a Teflon coating has since come on the market, but that was not available when I built my house

Some years later I heard another false rumor — this time that one side of the foil was coated with nickel.

I'm telling these stories because I've heard many such myths and misunderstandings over the years and they are usually told with great confidence by sincere people. One person's speculation is sometimes turned into a "fact," as it is passed on and gains a life of its own.

There is a German school of thought called Building Biology. Many of their teachings make sense, but I am deeply skeptical of their claims that houses be built without metal and that even in-floor heating systems should be avoided.

Some people do not feel well in a metal house, sometimes even a house with just a metal roof. Some of these problems are probably because of stray currents caused by faulty wiring or incorrect grounding. They can also be because the radiation from wireless gadgets inside the house bounces back from the metal walls (I have verified this with instruments). But there are a few cases where these explanations can be ruled out and it may be that the problem is simply that some people do not tolerate the metal itself in ways not yet understood. It may be that the metal disturbs the body's own electromagnetic field, or something else, but we don't know. I have myself observed that a steel floor seemed to give me symptoms, but I have visited several homes with metal walls and metal roofs without any problems, including my own home. There are presently 18 metal houses in the Snowflake EI community, and I have met dozens of people living in metal houses, so they seem to work well for the vast majority of people with EI. Building a house without steel can greatly increase the cost.

The most toxic material I had to use in the house was caulk. It takes a lot of caulk to build a modern house, especially in the bathroom and around the windows. I was told that "100% silicone" caulk was what people used, but there was no consensus on the most tolerable brand. They all offgassed eventually, but I wanted to find the best one for me.

I bought all the brands I could find in the three hardware stores in Kingman. I mail-ordered a phenol-based caulk from a store specialized in MCS equipment, and also found a special aquarium caulk.

I got a set of one-liter canning jars, which I washed and dried, so they were odorless. I put on my respirator and used a caulk gun to fully cover the insides of each canning jar with the various caulk samples, and labeled each jar with the name of the caulk and the date. Then this stinky collection was left in the open garage to offgas without lids on.

Every few days I sniffed each jar very cautiously, by using my hand to direct a tiny whiff of the fumes towards my nose. If I didn't smell anything, then I cautiously sniffed the jar directly.

The aquarium caulk was the clear winner. It was odorless within a couple of days. After two weeks the first of the regular caulks became inert. A week later the next was okay. Soon after that, the rest were fine, except one which took several months.

It was not surprising that the aquarium caulk was the best. Apparently regular caulks are so toxic that they can kill fish, hence the need for a special aquarium product. But the aquarium caulk cost many times more than regular caulk and I was doubtful it would hold up well in a sunny outdoor environment. It also came in small tubes that didn't fit into a caulking gun, so it was more work to use it. We only used this caulk in some places inside the house at the end of construction, and later for some maintenance.

The best of the regular caulks was used everywhere else inside the house, while the second-best was used on the outside. This was because the second-best caulk was significantly cheaper and should last longer in an outdoor environment.

The single most important choice when building an EI house is probably which paint to use, or whether to cover the walls with some other material instead, such as tile or foil.

With the large surface area of the walls and ceilings, even a slightly irritating material can be a big problem.

I have been inside several houses painted with "safe" paints that still bothered me several years after they were painted. I have seen several houses that have been ruined by using a paint not tolerated by the owner. This has happened when people assumed that a "non-toxic" or "zero VOC" paint was safe for them, or relied on word of mouth. I do not think there is any paint that works for everybody.

There were half a dozen "safe" paints available of various types. There were clay paints, milk paints, more regular formulations and even a joint compound called M-100 that can be used as a paint. The lineup of paints changes over time; some brands have since been added and others have disappeared.

I seemed to have more problems with the paints than most people with MCS, so I knew I had to be really careful with my choice. I knew from experience that I could never use one particular brand of "safe" paint, even though it was popular at the time.

I was very fortunate that I did well in my adviser's house even shortly after it was painted. I was really surprised that was even possible. That was a very good test. There was no doubt I should use the same paint, which was a home-made preservative-free clay paint.

It was great that I did not need to test all the candidate paints. That is a lot of work and takes months to complete. Here is what others have done: for each paint to test, buy a full 4x8 ft (2.5 x 1.3 m) sheet of drywall. Wrap the entire sheet in aluminum foil, so it is totally sealed and has no odor. Then paint the aluminum foil on one side of the sheet with the paint to be tested. Leave the sample to cure and air out for at least a month. If it seems odorless by then, then take the sheet inside the bedroom and place it close to the bed. This should be done when feeling the best, to see if it produces any symptoms.

Since I slept outside, I could not do this test anyway. I might instead have built a box to put my head in, and made sure the box itself did not produce any symptoms before sticking paint samples inside.

Some people have avoided paint entirely by having walls covered with glass, porcelainized steel, ceramic tiles, aluminum foil or aluminum wallpaper. Tiles and aluminum foil are the most popular alternatives. Tiling a whole house can be beautiful, but also very costly. Aluminum foil is cheap, but not so attractive, though people get used to it. Some people have hung decorative blankets on their aluminum walls.

There is a lot of tile in my house. All the floors are covered with tiles, and so are the walls and ceiling in the bathroom, as well as behind the kitchen counter to protect the clay paint on the wall. Tiles are mounted with a thinset that is mostly sand and cement and then the lines between the tiles are filled out with grout, which is also mostly sand and cement. Mounting tiles takes a lot of labor time. The building industry adds various chemicals to their pre-mixed thinsets and grouts that make it possible for unskilled laborers to slab on the tiles quickly, so a skilled tile setter is not needed. But some people do not tolerate these chemicals.

I once visited an MCS house where all the floors, walls and ceilings in the entire house had been covered with tile a few months earlier. They had used commercial thinset and grout and I could be inside only for a few minutes. It took well over a year before the owner could live there.

Someone told me about one brand of commercial thinset that had so few chemicals in it, that they were not listed on the Material Safety Data Sheet. I mixed up a sample in a big glass jar, let it sit for several days and then sniffed it. It stunk just like that all-tile house I just mentioned.

My adviser used a home-made thinset and grout in her house and so did I, despite the labor cost. There are recipes available on the internet.

There is a lot of drywall in a house, and I do not tolerate any brands of drywall, but it was fine once the walls were sealed. The seal is not perfect, so I still wanted the most tolerable drywall sheets I could get. I learned that they are made from mostly gypsum, with a brown paper backing. The gypsum can come from a mine, or it can be recycled from a demolished house or come from the filters of a coal-fired power plant. Gypsum that doesn't come from a mine can have various contaminants in it. Some factories also add formaldehyde or naphthalene to their gypsum. The brown paper backing is usually recycled paper.

The large manufacturers have several factories and several suppliers of their raw materials. In other words, each batch of the same brand can be very different. It did not make sense to test the brands ahead of time. I had to do it when it was time to order them for the house.

I know one person who offgassed all the drywall sheets for a year before installing them in his house. He did that in big stacks with spacers between each sheet. The drywall was used only for interior walls, so he didn't need to seal in any insulation.

I needed to use a cement board for the walls in the bathroom and for the window sills. I got a sample of the brand my adviser used, and it was inert. If I could afford it, I might have used cement boards on all the walls and ceilings, but sealing drywall sheets worked well enough. I briefly sniffed a sample of another major brand of cement board in the store and it had a solvent smell to it. I didn't try to air out a sample to see if it became inert later.

Magnesium oxide (MgO) boards had recently become available, but I was not interested in taking a chance with an unproven material. It has since been used in two houses in the area, one with great success, the other not. The problems may have been with a particular batch which was shipped from China. The quality controls are more lax over there and the shipment may also have been fumigated upon entry to the United States.

My adviser used formaldehyde-free fiberglass insulation in her house, and so did I. It is not a wonderful material, but it was fine inside the sealed walls.

When a group of people were building MCS houses in Snowflake in the 1990s, there was no formaldehyde-free fiberglass insulation available. The group contacted a small manufacturer of insulation and asked if they could make some without formaldehyde. The manufacturer responded that they were willing to try, if they could sell a full truckload of it. The group agreed and the manufacturer made the product, but it clogged up their machinery and created a big mess, so they said they would never do it again. The Snowflake group got what they needed and stored what they didn't use, which was later sold.

Some years later, more people were building houses in Snowflake. They contacted another manufacturer, who also agreed to try, with the same result.

Later on, the large manufacturer Johns Manville solved the production problems and offered the product to the general public. This is what I used. This product has been available on and off in the following years, sometimes only as blow-in insulation. There are other candidates, such as cellulose and magnesium oxide foams, though I have no experience with them. The Reflectix/Astro Foil aluminized "bubble wrap" products are widely used, but do not have the insulation value needed for a house (some people have tried and paid dearly in heating and cooling costs).

I bought a small roll of standard electrical wires of the ROMEX type that runs in every wall of a house. It had an odor I didn't like, so I rolled it out to bake in the sun. Even after a month I still found it unacceptable. This was a great surprise. I discovered that the roll I had was pre-greased to be easier to pull through electrical conduits. I got another brand and had no problems with it and just made sure to get the non-greased kind for the house.

My adviser had a steel/porcelain bathtub in her house, but there are few models available in that material, and I wanted a deeper model. The house in Dolan had an acrylic tub installed a couple of months before I moved in, and I did well with it. I decided acrylic was fine for me, I just made sure to offgas it before it was installed in the house.

I chose to use shower doors mounted on the edge of the tub. This is a great alternative to shower curtains that are made of stinky plastic or cotton that quickly becomes moldy.

The price of copper was rising and I heard that the building industry had embraced PEX tubing for water pipes. I didn't know of a single MCS house with PEX, but I decided to check it out.

I visited a plumbing firm in Kingman that had done work on MCS houses in Dolan. The owner was very helpful and told me his crew could install all the water pipes in a house in a single day with PEX, while it took them five days to do the same house with traditional copper. The PEX tubes are flexible and come in a roll with no need to solder a lot of small pieces of pipes together to get around corners. The other time-saving invention was the PEX fittings, that were either screwed together or crimped, which were a lot faster than soldering. PEX is clearly a lot cheaper than copper.

He gave me a sample of PEX and I bought some fittings to look at. I soaked the sample PEX tube and then tasted some water that had sat in it for a while. The PEX didn't impart much of a taste, and I knew that a biofilm eventually forms inside any water pipe, though I wondered about taking a shower in hot water from such a pipe.

Inspecting the fittings made me more concerned. These connections would be placed inside walls, where I had to trust that they would never ever leak, even decades later. A tiny leak will create mold, which could take me a long time to discover and possibly ruin the house. I also wondered if the PEX plastic might get brittle after a decade or two and crack around the crimps. The risk might be low, but the consequences very steep.

There didn't seem enough of a track record for me to trust PEX, so I didn't use it for the house water system. I did use it for most of the floor heating system with few fittings that could all be placed where they were visible for inspection. One of these fittings did leak. It would have been a mold disaster if it had happened inside a wall. It was a defective compression fitting with a pitted seat, which did not seal well enough around the PEX pipe.

A few years later there was a class-action suit against another manufacturer. The plaintiffs claimed that the fittings had leaked and damaged some houses. The suit was settled out of court.

In California there was a controversy about chemicals leaking into the drinking water and PEX was first legalized there in 2009.

There are many building products available with claims that they are "natural," "eco-friendly" or "green." These terms are vague and the products can still be very problematic for people with MCS.

Some products are made from recycled materials. That is otherwise a good idea, but I am leery about using recycled materials in my house since I wouldn't know where they came from and what contaminants are mixed in with them. Recycled concrete could come from a parking lot and may contain spilled motor oil. Drywall sheetrock with recycled gypsum could be contaminated with pesticides, fragrances and whatever else is in a regular building. A 2016 Danish study of new drywall sheets (see bibliography) found that all 13 samples they tested were contaminated with mold spores from the recycled paper backing. Recycled materials are worth so little that they are often stored improperly and allowed to become wet and moldy.

I've seen a brand of drywall sheets listed as an ecological product "made with 85% industrial byproducts." I assume that means it comes from the scrubbers on a coal-fired power plant, but I didn't look any further.

There are various "green" insulation products available. Cellulose insulation is usually made of recycled newspapers, with the accompanying concerns about the mold spores already present, besides the ink residue. Then there are the additives to prevent mold growth, to prevent fires and to keep the dust under control. Some products also have a glue added. About 15 to 25% of the product are these additives.

Another "green" insulation product is made of recycled denim, i.e. cotton. The product I looked into was 80% post-consumer denim, i.e. much of it would likely be contaminated with fabric softener, fragrances and other laundry chemicals. These chemicals are very difficult to wash out of the fabric again. Even if the denim is just scrap from a factory it may not be acceptable, since almost all makers of denim add a "signature fragrance." Wool is available for insulation. I haven't looked into that material, though I don't tolerate wool if it hasn't been washed several times. It may still be better than the formaldehyde-free fiberglass.

Some ecological products use non-toxic ingredients. That is laudable, but not necessarily tolerable. Linseed oil, citrus solvents, casein and other natural materials are non-toxic, but have a tendency to bother a lot of sensitive people.

I once visited a house built entirely of natural materials. The walls were made of straw bales, while the insides were covered with a wallboard made of straw that was pressed together without glue. The place smelled like a hay barn. The house was for rent and several people with MCS came to check it out, but it sat empty for years.

Just because something is natural doesn't mean it is safe for people with MCS. Turpentine used to be made from pine terpenes before it became cheaper to make it from petroleum. I used to be so sensitive to pine terpenes that I got dizzy just being near a pine forest on a hot day.

Sometimes the products that work best are terribly toxic with lots of VOCs that furiously outgas the first month or two, but then become more inert than the natural alternatives. There are people who prefer these kinds of paints in their houses, rather than natural paints that never seem to become completely odorless.

It is unfortunate that much of what is considered "green" or "ecological" is not really usable in an MCS house. Some of the products that do seem to work, such as rammed earth and plaster, are also costly to use. However much I'd like to use and promote recycled and natural products, my first priority was to build a house I could live in and afford.

My choice of materials will be further discussed in later chapters.

15. Planning for Off-Grid

My building site was five miles from the nearest utility service, so I needed to generate my own electricity with solar panels. Living off the grid was not a radical idea in that area which already had a medical clinic, a post office and at least a hundred homes off the grid. There were even two stores selling solar equipment.

Solar energy has interested me for a long time and in the early 1990s I visited several solar homes in Ohio and Wisconsin as part of various open-house tours. The technologies have advanced dramatically since these early solar homes, but many of the newer technologies are problematic for people with electrical hypersensitivities. The main problem is what is called an inverter, which converts the electricity from the solar panels into regular 110 volt AC electricity. It also sends out copious amounts of radio-frequency EMF and dirty electricity, which can turn the wires and solar panels into transmitting antennas. There are various designs of these inverters. I have tested each type with a Stetzer meter and an AM radio — they are all very problematic. The "optimizers" (also called Maximum Power Point Trackers) have the same problems.

I remembered those early solar pioneers and designed a similar system, using the 12 volt DC the solar panels provide, and not any inverter or optimizer.

Regular AC electricity cycles (alternates) sixty times a second, which means the EMF from the wires also cycles sixty times a second. DC electricity does not do this, and just has static fields around the wires, which I have no problem with.

It is a common misunderstanding that DC electricity is always benign — that is not true. DC electricity produced by a transformer, a battery charger or a car's alternator fluctuates and usually has high-frequency transients as well, thus the wires will radiate EMF. The same happens if a DC electrical motor or various electronics are used. The key to "clean" DC electricity is to use a steady source, i.e. solar panels and batteries, and be careful with what is connected to the system. Incandescent lights and some LED lights are "clean," while other LED lights and most electronics can create EMF and dirty electricity.

I had tinkered with small 12 volt solar systems before, including the one I was living with in Dolan, but I needed to scale it up for a whole house. Information about such "old technology" was scarce, but I got helpful information from two mail order companies catering to do-it-yourself off-grid folks. Even the obtuse *National Electric Code* had some useful information about low-voltage wiring and solar systems.

A 12 volt system is more complicated to build and use than grid power. It is necessary to estimate how much electricity is required and then calculate how many solar panels and batteries are needed. Because of the low voltage, the lengths of the wires in the house have to be minimized and thicker wires must be used. Once the system is built, it takes less maintenance than a car, but it is necessary to be aware of its limitations and live within them, as the electricity is not unlimited.

To adequately describe how to design and build such a solar system would take most of this book. Fortunately, such information is now available on the web at www.eiwellspring.org/offgrid.html.

My system is mostly used for 12 volt lights, and two small water pumps, but sometimes it also powers a 12 volt radio and a few other gadgets.

It is not realistic to do much cooking with 12 volt electricity. A regular hot plate uses 700–1000 watts, which is too much for a low-voltage system, but there are 12 volt crockpots available that work just like regular models. Mine consumes 100 watts and heats a can of food in an hour. The heating element does not send out EMF when powered by "clean" DC electricity.

I saw some articles about cooking with hydrogen in older issues of *Home Power* magazine. Hydrogen is the cleanest fuel of all and available from welding supply stores, so I wondered if I could use that to cook inside the house. It turned out that someone with MCS had already tried it, and it was still not odor free, so I gave up on that idea.

I considered solar cookers, and later bought one that I use to cook beans (it takes a whole day of full sun), but they cannot be the only cooking method.

I planned on continuing to cook outside, using a propane camping stove and a barbecue grill. I cook simple meals over a low fire, so I just needed to tend the pot a few times and didn't have to stay outside. Since I designed the house with the cooking area right outside the kitchen door, it is convenient enough to cook this way.

I needed a washing machine, but they use a lot of electricity and there are no 12 volt models available. I used a simple regular model that I connected to a propane generator. The generator also runs the well pump, which pumps water to a big holding tank.

I line-dried my laundry year-round in Dolan, but I was not sure it would work during the colder Snowflake winters. To be safe, I made sure to put an outlet for a clothes dryer in the outbuilding, so the generator could power it. I also looked into European centrifuges, as they use a lot less electricity — electricity from a generator is very expensive. Fortunately, I never needed to buy a dryer or centrifuge since line-drying the laundry works even in January, as long as it is a sunny day.

Another issue was the refrigerator. There were 12 volt models available, but I doubted I could tolerate the EMF and dirty electricity from the DC motor and electronics. Propane refrigerators have been available for about a century, but I did not want any propane inside the house. I solved that problem by designing a refrigerator closet on the side of the house, with a door I could easily access from the porch. The wall between the house and the propane closet was sealed airtight.

As a backup, I made it possible to have a 12 volt freezer or refrigerator in my outbuilding and power it from a separate solar system, but I never had to do that, as the propane refrigerator worked so well.

I designed the house around my off-grid needs. The cooking area had to be on the east side, so the house blocked the wind. Wind cools the pot — sometimes so much that it cannot boil, even with windbreakers around the stove. I also needed the kitchen right next to the outdoor cooking area, with a convenient door.

My access to the propane refrigerator, in its outside closet, had to be protected from rain and wind, and be convenient to the kitchen door. The wind protection was important, as a gust of wind can blow out the little pilot light in the refrigerator.

This all went together with having a covered porch that was protected from the wind, making it easy enough to come up with a house design that took care of all those needs.

I considered whether the cooking area should have a roof or not, for increased ventilation. I experimented on my porches in Dolan to see if cooking under a porch roof made any difference, and found it was better to not have a roof. It doesn't rain much in Arizona, and when it does the wall of the house usually creates a small rain shadow for the cooking area because of the wind direction, so a roof was not important.

This design has worked well for several years now. It is only about ten days a year where the weather prevents me from cooking outside.

The electrical system is designed to be simple to convert to use 110 volt AC electricity from an inverter or the grid, if it is ever extended out this far. I don't expect to ever need it, but it makes the house easier to sell.

Five other EI off-grid houses have since been built in my area. One has a setup very similar to my house.

Another house has two kitchens — a regular and a gas kitchen. The gas kitchen is in a corner of the house, with windows for cross-ventilation. The propane refrigerator has the burner encapsulated and vented directly to the outside. There is also a full-sized propane stove, that is placed in a vented glass box with doors on the front to access the stovetop and the oven.

Two other houses have very large solar systems, with inverters and enough 110 volt AC electricity to cook with, though they still have to run a generator when cooking on cloudy days. In one of these houses they spent a lot of money installing professional grade filters and shielded wiring, to greatly reduce the dirty electricity.

Living off the grid has benefits and drawbacks. It is not so much a pioneering effort any more, though we are still tinkering with ways to improve it for people who are environmentally sensitive. I have lived off the grid since 2008 and am quite satisfied, but it is not something everybody would like. My energy needs are a small fraction of the typical American household as I don't have air conditioning, garbage disposal, dishwasher or any always-on electronics, but I don't feel deprived. It also takes an open-minded electrician to install such a system, as the solar installers are no longer familiar with low-voltage DC solar systems.

16. Getting Started

The Dolan winters are mild, with January nights rarely below 30°F (-1°C). The 2007 winter was different, with the temperatures plummeting in mid-January. The first morning I measured 16° F (-9°C), while some low areas went down to 10°F (-12°C). We did not get above freezing the next day and the following night the temperature plummeted again. Old-timers said this was the coldest it had been since 1974.

Houses were not built for hard freezes in Dolan, so pipes froze and burst all over town during the second night. The town water supply could not keep up with all the leaks and was shut down for six days.

The pipes didn't break in my house, but with the water company shut down, I had no running water. I took water from the water heater to wash hands and flush the toilet, and used bottled water for cooking and drinking. Most of the other EI houses in Dolan had cisterns and I was welcome to shower there.

A friend I call Nevada-Jack was living in a travel trailer where all the pipes and the toilet bowl froze solid. Luckily, none of it broke.

I slept inside the house during the cold spell and did fine. The inside temperature was in the fifties (about 12°C), which apparently made what bothered me go dormant.

What was such an unusual cold spell for Dolan is routine for Snowflake. A burst water pipe can create serious mold in a house, so I made sure all pipes were well-protected in my house design. One thing I changed was that all the pipes in my outbuilding were mounted on the inside of the walls, instead of hidden in the walls. I think this saved them from freezing when Snowflake some years later saw temperatures down to −20°F (-30°C).

A stray cat showed up at my house the year before, while I was still unable to drive. He became a frequent guest and eventually hung around the house every day, even sleeping on my bed on the porch. A neighbor fed the cat the months I was away in Snowflake. I didn't expect to see him when I returned, but there he was, showing as much joy as a cat can. He obviously had lived in a loving home before he found himself on the streets of Dolan.

During this winter he wiggled into my sleeping bag to share the warmth every night. We had gotten attached to each other, so I decided it was best to take him with me to Snowflake.

The first part of construction was installing the septic sewage system. This could be done in the early spring without me present. Only after this has been installed and approved by the inspectors will the county accept an application for a building permit. I therefore needed it done well ahead of time.

I sent in the septic application and the percolation report early in the new year. It was good I was early, as it took months to get the permit. I had to call them several times to get it issued.

I hired the same contractor who did the digging work for the percolation test, as I really liked him. When he finally had the permit to start the work, he had a family emergency and was gone for three weeks, so the septic system was first installed and inspected in April. The delays were not a problem, as I first expected to start on the house in May. The contractor for the foundation was not available sooner, and it suited me fine to start camping in Snowflake in May, as April is cold and windy.

There was no road to my property. I had to build one from the nearest existing road, which was 1/3 mile (500 m) away. My new road had to go across a neighbor's land, using an easement. An easement is a legal right of way for a public road (or power line) to run along the edges of a private property.

I made sure there was such an easement before I bought the land, but the easement was blocked by a fence. There was no house on that property and the owner lived in another state. I contacted the owner, who was not interested in resolving the issue. I then talked to all sorts of county offices, which all agreed that a fence should not block an easement, but none of them wanted to help.

I then went to a real estate lawyer, who told me he saw a lot of neighbor conflicts over easements. He suggested I offered to pay to move the fence, as a much cheaper and less confrontational way to resolve the issue than any legal action. It seemed unfair that I had to pay the $2,400 it cost to hire a firm to move ¼ mile (400 meters) of fencing, but it was the best alternative, so that is what I did.

I had the fence moved, then a tractor bladed the new road and later on I had gravel put on it. The county issued a name for the road and a street number for my house.

This whole process took some months, with most of it happening while I was still in Dolan.

Spending the winter in Dolan impacted my health. My sensitivity to light and to my car had gotten worse and I knew I needed to be as strong as possible for managing the building project during the coming summer, I therefore decided to get some of the treatments in Dallas that had helped me two years before.

It took me five days to make it to Dallas, with one day of rest in Rodeo, New Mexico. I had to stop and rest every twenty minutes along the way. While I drove along the border in New Mexico the Border Patrol found my stops suspicious and had a patrol car there every time I stopped. The patrolmen were very polite, but I was glad to be free of them when I reached El Paso.

It was a little early to start a road trip in late March, but the weather cooperated most of the time. The exception was a big hailstorm that came while I spent a weekend at a friend's house outside Dallas.

On weekdays I stayed at a campground by Hickory Creek north of Dallas. There I noticed a vintage Airstream travel trailer with the stark "MCS look." I simply walked up to the woman and asked if she knew Dr. Rea. She replied that she had seen him that very morning. Dallas can be a small world if you know what to look for.

I headed home again after two weeks in Dallas. The treatments helped and the drive home went much easier.

I intended to spend the whole summer and fall in Snowflake while my house was built. I would be living in a tent with the expectation of heading back to Dolan in early November. I hoped the project could then get finished over the winter, without me being there.

Now that I was back from Dallas, I was ready to move to Snowflake for the summer as soon as the contractor was ready to start on the foundation. He had promised me to start in early May, but he was busy and kept delaying into June.

I was getting nervous that we might start so late in the year that I could not leave the project to continue on its own by November, so I called a few other contractors to see if they could start sooner. Some replied that they would not work with additive-free concrete; one was willing to do it, but he wanted $3,000 extra. For that price he said he also guaranteed there would be no oil spills from his equipment.

Finally, my original contractor gave me a semi-firm starting date. I immediately sent in the application for the building permit, and two weeks later I moved to Snowflake.

I delayed sending in the application until then, as I knew the county penalized people who didn't start building soon after it was issued. The county office told me they now issued the permits within days, so it should be safe to run it tighter. I also wanted to be able to deal with any problems in person, and there was a problem as the inspector interpreted their new building code differently than I did regarding a gray-water system. The inspector made this impossible to do, but I appealed to the county engineer who enthusiastically agreed with my point of view.

I needed an insurance policy to cover me against fire, theft and if a worker fell off the roof (which nearly happened). I did that with a homeowner's insurance policy, but it took some legwork to find someone willing to insure me. Most of the insurance companies would not insure a house that was more than ten miles from a fire station. One didn't like that there was no grid-connected electricity (no idea why). It was also an issue that the house wasn't built yet and I wasn't a licensed general contractor. But I found a local agent who was rather new in business, and he saw no problem taking me on. He just asked me to call him once the house was finished so he could go out and take a picture for his files.

I bought a small flat-bed trailer that my car could comfortably pull. This allowed me to haul a lot of materials myself, saving me a lot of money. The large or heavy loads still had to come by delivery truck.

I also had a second phone installed at my friend's house, so I could easily call the contractors and suppliers, and they could leave me voice mails.

The summer before, I noticed two concrete slabs in the yard where I was camping. My friend told me that some years ago a homeless man with MCS wanted to live there in two garden sheds. He had the two slabs poured, but then abandoned the project. Now I used one slab for an 8x10 (2.5x3 m) steel garden shed I bought and hauled on my new trailer. It came as a kit, which took two days to erect.

The shed was offgassed within three weeks. I installed some metal shelving, a small folding table and a steel chair. It then became my storage space and living room for the next six months. I continued to sleep in my tent, but now I didn't need to store clothes and camping gear in my car, and I had a comfortable space to hang out and not be in anyone's way.

My friends rolled their eyes when I showed up with a cat, but he quickly charmed everybody. I had a cat door installed on the shed that was his safe place to sleep during the day, while he slept in my tent at night. He quickly adapted to his new home.

17. The Foundation

The foundation we built is called a stem wall system with a floating concrete floor. This type of foundation was necessary for the radiant floor heating. I chose radiant floor heating because it allowed me to heat the house without any air ducts, noise, fumes or EMF in the house. It works by circulating hot water through pipes embedded in the concrete floor, and is the most comfortable way to heat a house. The downside is that it needs the more expensive foundation.

Since the whole concrete floor is heated, it is warmer than it otherwise would be and must be well-insulated to prevent excessive heat loss. I know one MCS house where they did not insulate the concrete floor, resulting in a heating bill they could not afford. They had to use portable electric heaters instead. This was even in an area with mild winters. I am saying this because there are some people who believe it is not necessary to fully insulate the floor slab.

We had to insulate the heated floor both along the sides and down towards the soil. We used insulating foam boards that were able to carry the weight of the floor.

A low concrete wall was built on the perimeter of the house, called a stem wall. This stem wall was insulated with the foam boards on the inside and protected the heated floor from the elements. The outer walls of the house were later built on top of the stem wall.

An added benefit of the stem wall was that we could then keep the floor at least five inches (12 cm) above the porch and surrounding soil. This gives some protection against termites and flooding, both of which can ruin the house for people with MCS.

It is customary in Arizona and several other states to protect houses against termites by soaking the soil with pesticides before the house is built. In some areas it is required by the building code. The inspectors will often allow a builder to not poison the soil if there is a specific health issue, but I know of one house where they refused to accommodate. The owner had to build the house entirely without wood to satisfy the inspectors. This might have been a good choice anyway, since an older MCS house nearby did get a termite infestation some years later.

Termites were less of a problem in the area I built. None of the EI houses in Snowflake have been pesticided for termites and there have been no problems.

I met with the foundation contractor out on my land a week before he started. I had staked the four corners of the house one evening, where I could use the North Star to find true north, since proper orientation is important for a solar house. (Compasses do not show true north in Western America and I couldn't remember the correction factor.) The contractor checked to make sure the stakes fit the dimensions on the drawings and that the corners were all squared. Then he put in his own markers.

We broke ground on June 20, 2007. The contractor arrived with three helpers and a tractor. The tractor bladed my driveway and the new road into my property, while the contractor did his last measurements and setups using a laser leveler. Then the tractor used its backhoe to dig a trench along the perimeter of the house where the stem wall was to be built.

Steel rebar was laid in the bottom of the trench and then it had to be inspected before we could continue.

I had registered my new road with the county months before, but it did not yet appear on their printed maps or any GPS navigators. I gave the inspector's office a map so they could find the building site, but the inspector didn't bring the map and could not find us. I called the inspector late in the afternoon, when he was back in the office, to give him directions and make sure he knew about the map.

The next day it was a different inspector, and he didn't bring the map either — again no inspection.

The third day we finally had the inspection. It was a third inspector, who brought the map and had no problems finding his way. He also seemed friendlier and more open minded than some of the inspectors, so I asked him how they were dispatched and from then on made sure it was him who did the inspections. There were no further problems with the inspections and this inspector was actually helpful with information later on. The county has since had a large turnover of their inspectors, and none of those involved in my project work there anymore. There were a total of nine inspection visits at various stages of the construction, including the final inspection at the end.

With the inspection done, we could finally continue. The next morning a 35-ton six-wheel-drive concrete truck came and poured concrete into the dug trenches. The contractor then continued building up the stem walls with hollow-core concrete blocks, which he cemented together. It was hot work sitting there in the relentless summer sun, so he started each morning at 5 a.m.

The contractor needed some water for the masonry work and brought a big plastic drum he filled from a cattle watering tank a couple of miles away.

After the stem walls were built, a concrete truck came and filled the hollow blocks, so we now had an eight-inch (20 cm) thick solid wall around the perimeter of the house. The floor of the house eventually became level with the top of this low wall.

Once the stem wall was finished, it looked like a big storage bin. Then it was time to fill the "bin" with gravel. Dump trucks brought in gravel they deposited in a big pile next to the house. The contractor made sure that the gravel was clean and came directly from a gravel pit. A load of gravel for another MCS house once arrived contaminated with diesel fuel and had to be sent back. Some gravel companies deliver recycled gravel, which can have all sorts of contaminants.

An oversized "Bobcat" (actually made by Case) with a bucket on the front transferred the gravel to the "bin" surrounded by the low stem wall. Layer after layer was added and compacted, while slowly building up the foundation for the floor of the house. This build-up had to be done slowly, so there would be minimal settling. Otherwise the floor would eventually crack.

Water was needed for compacting the gravel and since I had no well yet the contractor rented a water trailer to haul water from a spigot fourteen miles (22 km) away. I could have saved the thousand dollars this cost me, if I had the well drilled early, but I had not understood that a lot of water was needed this early in the project. My advisor used a very long irrigation hose to bring water to her building site from a neighbor, but that was not possible in my case.

There was no shade on the building site, but now I had learned to protect myself enough against the sun to allow me to be there for a few hours despite my light sensitivity. I felt fine wearing two layers of the sun protective clothing, a hat with a very wide brim, a sun mask, non-toxic titanium sunscreen and some really dark (2%) sunglasses.

I made sure to be present whenever heavy equipment was in use. It was fascinating to watch the contractor expertly directing with hand signals, as if he conducted a symphony orchestra.

The other reason I had to be present was to watch out for mistakes, as heavy equipment can create a big mess in a hurry. I once had to stop a delivery truck from driving over a low escarpment because the driver was too lazy to back up. A few times I was able to spot a problem in time, such as when the crew forgot to make a hole in the stem wall for the sewage pipe to later pass through.

I hired the sub-contractor with the big "Bobcat" to extend and upgrade the jeep trail going into the area. He switched the bucket out with a big blade and off he went. Within a couple of hours, he had bladed two miles of dirt road. Now I had a primitive road giving me a much more direct path to town and the EI neighborhood. It has since served me well, as long as it is dry.

With the house gravel bed built up, it was then time for the plumber to install the water and sewage pipes that run below the floor. He had promised to work on a certain day, but then he got a well-paid job in some fancy house. The foundation contractor called the plumber daily, and each time was promised the work would be done the next day, but it took three days before the plumber actually showed up.

The foundation contractor was not able to do any other work until the plumber had done his, and he did not have any one-day jobs lined up. He was paid for the whole foundation job and it was he who hired and paid the plumber, so the delay was therefore his responsibility. He was not happy losing three days of work.

The plumber interpreted my drawings incorrectly and placed the drain to the bathtub six inches off. Nobody caught the mistake in time, so my bathroom ended up six inches wider than planned. This was not a problem, but it could have been. It is best not to draw a house with the assumption that everything is built so precisely. Walls and corners can easily be an inch or two off.

The plumber also nearly made another mistake, but I caught that one in time. I later had to fire him and hire another plumber to do the sewage line outside the house. His little trencher was not strong enough to handle the rocks. He then tried to put the sewage line in a sweeping half-moon-shaped trench, which is not a good idea.

It pays to watch out for shoddy work. I have a friend whose septic tank was installed backwards. The contractor covered up his error, rather than correct it. This caused endless problems once the house was occupied. My friend eventually had to install a whole new septic system, at her own cost.

With the under-slab pipes in place, the contractor installed a strong membrane of 6 mil (0.15 mm) plastic on top of the gravel. This membrane blocks any radon gas and prevents moisture from wicking up through the concrete floor.

Rigid foam insulation boards were then placed on top of the membrane, to insulate the warm floor from the soil. Foam boards were also placed on the inside of the stem wall. These boards didn't stink, but might still contain flame retardants and other chemicals. They were too costly to use in the rest of the house, anyway.

The foam boards were not available locally, the contractor had to drive the 200 miles (320 km) to Phoenix to pick up a load of them. That was an unexpected extra cost.

Rebar was then installed on top of the foam boards, to reinforce the concrete slab that was soon to be poured. Half-inch (1.25 cm) PEX tubing was then placed on top and tied to the rebar, so the tubes could not float up when the concrete was poured. These tubes were later used to heat the floor with hot water.

The standard thickness of such a slab is four inches (10 cm). We made it five inches thick to increase the thermal mass, which helps keep the house cool in the summer and works with the solar heating system to warm the house on winter nights.

Then it was time for Big Concrete Day. It was mid-July and the contractor wanted the concrete to set before the sun got really hot, so we started at 6 a.m. I had gotten a bad EMF exposure a few days before and was not able to drive my car, but I didn't want to miss this exciting event. Fortunately, a friend volunteered to drive me out there despite the early hour.

It was a spectacle well worth seeing. Two concrete trucks, two drivers and three contractors worked furiously to get the concrete distributed and smoothed out before it set. It all went well, and now the floor of the house was in place.

Some contractors pour diesel fuel on a finished concrete slab, to make it look nicer. This happened with one MCS house built years ago. They tried all sorts of ways to get the diesel out, but it had soaked into the concrete and was impossible to remove. They finally had to seal it with a membrane and pour a new concrete slab over it, which solved the problem. The membrane was a product called Aluseal, consisting of heavyweight aluminum foil with plastic on both sides (a plastic membrane alone would not contain the diesel).

My contractor knew he was building an environmental house and he didn't do anything toxic. He also made sure that we used concrete without any chemical additives. Modern concrete usually contains various additives (called admixtures) to make the concrete stronger, frost resistant, faster to cure and easier to work with. Some companies even add fly ash and biocides to their concrete. These additives can all be a problem for people with MCS.

Using admixture-free concrete meant it could not be poured during a hard freeze and it had to be wet cured. Wet curing is not commonly done any more and some contractors charge extra or simply refuse to do it. Wet curing seemed simple enough: the concrete was covered by plastic sheeting, to keep it moist, and after three days the sheeting was pulled off.

The only mishap was during a break, when I stood and talked with the contractor. I suddenly heard a buzzing sound, like an angry bee passing close to my head. One of the hired hands had walked a hundred yards away to do a little target practice. The bullet hit a rock and then ricocheted right past my head. Guns are almost an everyday item in rural Arizona. When the house was later framed a rattlesnake came out from the pile of lumber and headed for the worksite, but one of the contractors shot it with the gun he kept on the dashboard of his car.

Houses without radiant floor heat can use a much simpler and cheaper foundation than the stemwall system I used. Many EI houses in Arizona use a monopour foundation instead. This kind of foundation has no masonry work and can be built in just a few days. The whole foundation is simply one big concrete slab, which extends out under the exterior walls. The downside is that it can't be insulated as well as with a stem wall and the floor tends to be closer to the soil. Forms have to be used when pouring the concrete and contractors commonly grease the forms with diesel fuel that can soak into the edges of the concrete. This can be avoided by supplying the contractor with vegetable oil, or pay extra to use disposable forms.

It took three weeks to build the foundation. Now we just needed the concrete porches and the slabs for the shed and the generator. I paid the contractor for the work, so he had cash to do the final part, but his bank insisted on holding the money for two weeks, before he could draw the money. This delayed the remaining concrete work and thus the start of the framing. I had to call the framers and tell them to come two weeks later and also had to delay a truckload of lumber.

The delay was actually welcome. It had rained almost every afternoon during July and it tapered off once we got into August, so my house was barely rained on before the roof was on. I wanted the lumber to be kept as dry as possible. It was also good to have some time off before the most hectic period of the project.

18. Building the Shell

With the foundation finished, a new set of contractors moved in, and I became more involved in the project.

I took care of ordering the materials including calling and visiting the suppliers and arranging transport of the materials. This is normally done by a general contractor, but can also be done by the owner/builder, unless the bank requires a professional general contractor.

The materials stream was a balancing act. If they arrived too early, then they could be in the way, get moldy or even get stolen, and if they came too late then the contractors had nothing to do.

I had some project management experience and a technical education, which was helpful, though I had no experience with house construction. With the guidance of my adviser and the excellent people I hired as contractors, I was able to do my part.

The main contractor and my adviser gave me an approximate timeline for the project and told me in what order the major deliveries of materials were needed. I checked with the vendors of trusses, steel panels, windows, etc., to find out what their delivery schedules were, so I could keep the contractors supplied with a steady flow of materials.

In most cases the vendors could deliver with two weeks' notice. One told me they had been so backed up the year before it took them eight weeks to deliver their trusses.

During the previous month I had prepared myself by visiting the vendors in the area, including six hardware and building supply stores, two plumbing supply stores, two electrical supply stores and a truss manufacturer. They carried a variety of products and had widely varying prices and quality of service. Some of the stores catered to professional builders, but only one of them told me they were not interested in my business.

I surveyed the four lumberyards. One was the store that didn't want my business. Two stored their lumber outdoors, which I didn't like, as that increased the risk that the lumber was moldy and warped.

I established a good relationship with a particular person at the contractor's desk at my chosen lumberyard. She took the time to understand my special needs and kept an eye on what was coming to the store. She was very helpful during the framing of the house, when I needed extra lumber in a hurry, and much preferably the less-odorous kind. She was very good, and it was no surprise that she was soon promoted out of that job. I bought most of my materials in this store. I was highly visible with my respirator, so the staff noticed I was there a lot and I got great service throughout the store. Even years later some of the staff greeted me warmly.

In some stores I told them I was building a whole house and asked for their contractor's discount. Some agreed while some only had discounts on large orders. The discounts I got saved me at least a thousand dollars.

I got good service at most of the stores, even when I asked if we could go outside to discuss something, so I could take my respirator off.

Only one store had poor service. I had to hang over the counter at the pro desk for several minutes, before the staff would "notice" me, even if they were not busy. That was hard, as they had three computers sitting on the counter. If I stood back a few feet, the staff never "saw" me. The entire pro-desk staff was gone within the year, and the store closed some years later.

One small hardware store was the most difficult place to be inside, even with my respirator on. But the staff was used to people with MCS and very helpful to us. One day I walked in there the air quality was so bad I had to hurry out immediately. A staffer saw me and came out to say that they just had a paint spill inside. They were very helpful and brought out what I needed.

I gave a hand-drawn map to each of the two stores I got materials delivered from, so their drivers could find my building site. They had no problem finding us. Some of the materials, such as the windows and doors, I could transport on my own trailer.

The first thing we built was a steel garden shed, like the one I was living in. It was 10x14 ft (3x4 m), which is the largest size that did not require a building permit in Navajo county. The shed was very handy to store various materials during construction, and also later on.

The other reason for the shed was that I could live in it for the rest of the summer, if I wore out my welcome camping in my friend's yard. Then I would buy a portable camping toilet, a small water tank and a super-insulated cooler to get by with. Fortunately, I was welcome in my friend's yard for the duration.

We started framing in mid-August. The contractor gave me a list of what lumber he needed and I took it to my chosen lumberyard. They entered it into their computer and gave me an estimated price. It was astronomical. I had ordered mostly Douglas fir, with a few pieces of redwood. They had entered it all as redwood, which cost fifteen times more!

I signed up for the store's credit card, which gave me 10% off the first purchase. I used this discount for the lumber package. At this point I was flush with cash, so I paid off the credit card and didn't waste any money on interest.

It took two weeks to frame the house. It happened at a furious pace, with two workers using nail guns and a third worker cutting and feeding them lumber. It took only two days before the contractor gave me a list of more lumber to get and I had to order another truck delivery. It was like trying to feed an insatiable monster — more sticks, more sticks!

I drove to the work site every day during this hectic period to see if they had any questions or needed more materials. I typically stayed for half an hour and then went back to make phone calls or continued on to a lumberyard. It was the busiest part of the project because we needed the house framed and closed in against the rain as fast as possible.

Professionally managed projects run at this pace all the way through, but my health could not hold up for that. Just these few weeks took their toll.

We used Douglas fir to frame the house, as that is somewhat less aromatic than pine, and it was available at a similar cost. The lumberyard normally doesn't distinguish among the types of wood they sell for studs, as long as they are strong enough, but my contact there was looking out for me. She also made sure all our lumber was kiln dried, so it was less likely to be moldy or warped.

The wood we used was still aromatic, and I don't really know if this extra effort made any difference once the walls were sealed.

The bottom plate in the walls needs to be mold resistant, as it can be moist there due to condensation against the cold floor. Moisture can also linger there if flooding ever happens, such as from a leaky pipe. The standard material is pressure treated wood, but that is toxic, so we used redwood instead, which is extremely durable and rot resistant. It is very aromatic, but it was not a problem when the walls were sealed.

We did not use steel studs in the outer walls, as that would dramatically reduce the insulation and possibly cause condensation on the attached drywall. It is vital to avoid condensation, as it encourages mold growth.

The framing was done like an ordinary house. I could have used any framing crew, though I'd have to make sure they didn't smoke while working to avoid butts left inside the wall cavities. The only thing a little unusual was that the walls were double-framed with staggered studs. This eliminated a lot of thermal bridging and gave room for ten inches (25 cm) of insulation instead of the typical six inches (15 cm). This is not a special EI building method, though many modern super-insulated houses now use pre-fabricated SIPs (Structurally Integrated Panels) instead. I didn't use SIPs because they contain a lot of glue, even the formaldehyde-free versions.

Once the walls were framed, they were covered with house wrap. This is a type of plastic that slows down air movement on a windy day, but allows the walls to breathe. This is very important, as the innermost part of the walls were later sealed with a moisture barrier. There can be only one moisture barrier in a wall — if there are two, moisture can be trapped inside and cause mold and rot.

Horizontal lumber was then nailed to the outside wall to hold the house wrap in place and for the siding to be screwed onto later. Wooden sheathing (plywood or OSB) are used for that purpose in regular construction, but they are too toxic. We used 1x4 (2.5x10 cm) lumber, spaced 2 ft (60 cm) apart.

The trusses were custom built of lumber by a local firm. They designed the trusses from the house plans I gave them, which was simple enough. The trusses were made a few days in advance and delivered the day before we needed them, so they did not sit around on the work site.

I hired a crane to lift the trusses in place and had the three workers nail the trusses down. I called the crane operator the evening before to make sure he was coming and learned that his old rig had a breakdown, and he could not come. He suggested another crane operator, whom I called right away. The second crane operator said he was booked up for several days, but if we agreed to start early and hurry up, he could fit me in the next morning.

The crane arrived early the next morning and it took less than two hours of intense work to get the trusses in place before the crane could hurry on to the next job.

The three framers then continued nailing 2x4 (5x10 cm) lumber horizontally across the trusses so it looked like a giant ladder. These horizontals are called purlins.

The steel roofing was screwed on top of the purlins. It took the three-man crew four hours to install them all. It was the simplest roof possible, with just two big surfaces. A more complicated roof would cost more and have more places where leaks can develop.

We used 26 gauge Pro-Panel steel sheets that were painted and pre-cut at the factory in Colorado before they were delivered to the work site. These types of panels create a very strong and durable roof that is virtually maintenance free for several decades. There are various other brands available which have been used on other MCS houses.

This roofing system is commonly used on barns and industrial buildings in America. Many homes in Europe have roofing tile mounted on purlins. American homes are usually built differently, using toxic plywood and shingles. Instead of the purlins, plywood is mounted on top of the trusses where it creates a "deck," which is then covered with a waterproof membrane. Roof shingles or steel panels are then mounted on top of that.

The oldest MCS house in the neighborhood with such a plywood-free roof was built in 1988 and it is still sound thirty years later.

I continued to schedule the same open-minded building inspector. He was not familiar with this roofing system, but he saw no problem with it. I didn't even need to show him the brochure from the manufacturer. I have since heard of other inspectors who refused to approve what they were not familiar with. The builders then had to use toxic plywood which usually went okay if they sealed the ceiling well. Others avoided the plywood by building the "deck" with wooden planks.

My house now had a roof and house wrap to provide protection against rain. That was a relief, since it was still monsoon season and I didn't want the lumber to be wet more than absolutely necessary. The framing went so fast that we had only two showers before the roof was on.

Next came the exterior doors. We used steel doors that had small strips of wood along the edges and foam-core insulation. They came with an off-white primer coating, so they could be painted any color.

We used the same type of door inside the house as well, and we didn't paint any of them. I bought all the doors at the same time and left them outside to roast in the sun to let them offgas. They were placed on scraps of wood, so they were not touching the ground.

It took a couple of months before the interior doors were needed, so they sat outside long enough that sand drifted up along the edge of one door. The sand was moist from rain, and mold started to grow where the sand touched the wooden edge of the door. When I discovered the mold, it was too late to remove it and the door had to be discarded.

We used double-glazed windows with aluminum frames. Aluminum frames never need to be painted and are odorless, but not as well insulated as vinyl or wooden frames. Most aluminum frames are not insulated, but we used the kind with a built-in thermal break, which makes a big difference.

In another EI house, there was an ordering error where they got the windows without the thermal break, and the error was not caught in time. They continue to have problems with condensation around the windows every winter. The condensation gathers on the window sill and sometimes makes the drywall around the window wet.

Windows can be ordered with low-E glass, which increases the insulation of the window and makes it reflect some of the sunlight. I didn't want low-E glass on the south windows, which I needed to catch the heat of the winter sun, but I wanted low-E glass on the three other sides of the house. The sales clerk made a mistake and entered the order for all the windows without low-E glass. I didn't catch the error when I approved the order on a printout, and the windows were made to order, so they could not be returned. I had to pay for the whole order and then order the missing windows. I used two of the "surplus" windows in the outbuilding, and I gave one window to a local community center where it is now their kitchen window.

The store clerk forgot to send off the second window order. I first discovered the mistake when I called two weeks later, to see if the windows had arrived.

These two mistakes caused a delay of three weeks before I had all the windows. There were other things the contractors could work on, but I had to stop construction for a week while waiting for the last windows. This break was very welcome. I would have had to stop work very soon anyway because I was too exhausted. Twice it made me so sick I had to lie down for a day to rest and some days I was able to only drive the car for 15 or 20 minutes at a time. It was painful to use the telephone. People told me I tended to tell them the same story several days in a row. I urgently needed a week off. The contractors didn't mind, either.

The siding was the same type of steel panels we used for the roof, just with thinner (29 gauge) material. They were custom cut at the factory which meant I could first order them once the house was framed and we could measure the exact sizes. (The exact length was not critical for the roof panels, which could be ordered before the trusses arrived.) The delivery was a day late with the crew standing idle waiting for the delivery truck to arrive.

The windows had to be installed before the siding, so some panels had to wait until the missing windows arrived.

The manufacturer forgot to include a bag of their color-matching screws, but they quickly sent them by express mail. I was able to borrow some of these special screws meanwhile.

The steel siding went on fast. The panels were mounted with screws to horizontal pieces of wood that were mounted to the wall studs. It took a lot more time to put in the trim pieces around the windows, the bottom of the walls, the edges of the roof, the soffits, etc.

The contractor put copious amounts of caulk around the windows, as I wanted to be absolutely sure no water could seep into the wall, which had happened in some earlier houses.

I purchased a roll of "flat stock" steel that matched the pre-cut panels in color. This was used to make custom pieces of trim and to wrap any remaining exposed wood, such as the beam under the porch roof, posts, door frames, etc. I wanted all exterior wood encased in steel to avoid the need for any paint.

It takes a lot of time to custom cut and bend pieces of metal. I was keenly aware that we still had lots to do before I had to return to Dolan for the winter, consequently we deferred some of this trim work until the next summer.

It was now early fall and my house was fully enclosed against the elements. It looked like it was almost done, but in reality, we were only halfway there.

19. The Well System

I continued to live in my friend's yard, sleeping in my tent and using the garden shed as living room and storage space for my belongings. Even though I had offgassed my tent by hanging it from the rafters in my Dolan garage for two years, it still smelled of plastic when sitting in the sun, but was fine at night.

I had to take the tent down every morning to protect it from the sun's ultraviolet rays. It took only a few minutes to do, and I saved some time by leaving the large sand stakes in the ground every day.

A handful of people passed through the area over the summer on their quest for a safe house to rent. Two of them had also visited us the previous year. This year one of them found a rental in Dolan Springs and moved in right away. The other still had no luck.

When I moved out of my rental house in Dolan Springs the following year, that house became a stepping-stone for more people trying to settle in Arizona.

Sometimes there were visitors from the other communities in Arizona, giving us a good occasion for a small party. With multiple houses going up, construction was a popular topic of conversation and during one party someone made a song using the melody from the Beatles song "Yellow Submarine." The refrain was "we all live in a Pro-Panel house," referring to the steel panels used on most of the houses.

One visitor came with a Toyota Prius hybrid car. This is essentially an electric car with a gasoline-powered electric generator. I was curious about these types of cars and drove it once around the circular driveway for about twenty seconds. Even this short drive affected me so thoroughly that my brain felt really strange for the rest of the day and evening.

With the house construction becoming less intensive, I was able to begin on the well system, which was gradually installed over the next couple of months.

The well driller came out to look at the site and I showed him where I wanted the well to be, which was fine with him. A few days later he came back with a big drill rig and a tanker truck filled with soapy water. It takes a lot of water to cool the drill and flush out the loosened material. The well driller was used to MCS customers and used a non-toxic dish detergent as lubricant in the water.

The drill rig started with a roar and a dust cloud from the sandy topsoil, and continued for two days until the drill hit the aquifer 320 ft (100 m) below the surface. The water was under so much pressure that it briefly gushed up the bore hole like a geyser.

The well casing was installed and the pump lowered into the hole. This type of pump is placed deep in the well, below the waterline, where it pumps water up to the surface through a long pipe. I had the choice of steel and PVC pipes, and chose PVC. This choice may surprise some readers, but I saw the badly corroded steel pipes pulled out of a nearby well and didn't want my drinking water to come through such a pipe.

If my house was connected to the grid, I would have a small pressure tank that the well pump automatically fills whenever needed. A person living in the house might not even notice when this happens.

Since my house was off the grid, my system was more complicated. A regular well pump uses a lot of electricity when it runs and I did not have that available on demand, as a grid-tied house does. I had four main choices: a solar pump, a wind pump, a wind powered bubble-pump and a generator-powered pump. There are many issues to consider, such as cost, maintenance, longevity, water pollution and EMF, which would take a whole chapter to cover fully.

The wind pumps have served the American West for well over a century and are still manufactured by Dempster and Aermotor. I'd like to own one, just because I love looking at them, and they are totally EMF free. The solar pumps are the new kings on the range, but they tend to radiate a lot of EMF from the long wire into the well. I visited one that made my AM radio crackle even 150 ft (50 m) away.

The bubble-pumps were enticing, but I was told they pollute the water with tiny amounts of oil.

I installed my well a hundred yards from the house, so a solar pump can be safely installed in the future, but I simply did not have the money to install a solar or wind pump. I went with the generator pump, which was much cheaper, since I needed a generator anyway.

The generator option uses the same type of well pump as used for a grid-tied house, but the pump is only run weekly with power from a generator. The washing machine is run at the same time, also using power from the generator.

I later learned that jack pumps, the type usually seen in oil fields, are also available in small solar models suitable for off-grid homes.

All the well pump options available to me delivered water intermittently, so they all required a storage tank. In the old days, ranches had water towers to deliver water to the house by gravity pressure, but this is not common today. I placed my water tank on a little knoll next to the well so water runs to the house by gravity. The pressure is barely enough to flush the toilet, and too low to take showers, so a solar-powered 12 volt RV-style booster pump increases the water pressure to a normal level. A small 20-gallon (76 liter) pressure tank buffers the booster pump.

Many of the houses in Dolan used plastic tanks that gave the water a slight smell. I was also concerned about algae growth, which is promoted by light, so I wanted a steel tank. Shortly after I arrived in Snowflake a local shop that built steel tanks to order was short on work. They built a popular tank model and placed it in front of the local grocery store with a FOR SALE sign on it. I bought it at a good price. They delivered it to my yard, where it sat for months before it was time to install.

It was a big, 3000-gallon (11,000 liter) tank with round sides. They left it on its side, on a slight incline, so I was concerned the wind might make it roll downhill. I put a concrete block under it on the downhill side, and thought the problem was fixed, but later a strong wind gust sent the tank rolling *uphill* and then back right over the block. I was lucky there was no damage.

Two non-EI neighbors were not so lucky. They both had their plastic water tanks taken away and destroyed by high winds — one of the tanks rolled for miles across the desert and was never found again. My neighbors were careless and didn't keep enough water in the tanks to weigh them down.

Once my well was installed, I contracted with the tank builder to install the tank and pipes down towards the house. I stipulated in the contract that I must be present, and we scheduled the work for the following Monday. I happened to go out to the worksite on Friday, and there the crew was at work installing the tank! It was good I was there, as I realized we needed a shut-off valve.

The contractor insisted on supplying his own materials, so he could earn a markup. I thought that was alright, until he billed me $85 for the valve, which I could buy at a local store for $24 — a 250% markup.

The contractor brought a backhoe, which was used to hoist the steel tank in place and dig the trenches. They laid an underground pipe down to a convenient spot next to the garden shed, where they installed a hydrant, as the line could not yet be extended to the house. They also laid the underground electrical cable to the generator, which I later installed on a concrete pad next to the shed.

I hired a teenager to climb down into the water tank and scrub it before we started using it. The house building contractor then used his generator to fill the tank, so he had water for his projects and the tank was firmly weighed down against any storms. I delayed buying my own generator until the following year to defer the expense and avoid the risk of theft.

The tank leaked a little at a seam, but the tank-builder came out and fixed that with a welder.

I sent a sample of the well water to be tested at a laboratory. It showed no pesticides or other chemicals. There was no arsenic and acceptable amounts of various minerals, such as manganese, magnesium and iron. Several wells in the area had such high levels of iron that they use water softeners and even special iron filters. Such filters use up a lot of water and water costs more when pumped with a generator, so I was glad I didn't need them.

I later installed a sediment filter, and the water tank acted as a settling tank. I just had to change the sediment filter four times a year and flush out the gunk at the bottom of the water tank once a year.

We now had water available, though it had to be carried from the outdoor hydrant in buckets.

It was the following summer that the house was finally connected to the water line, as the line had to go through the outbuilding before it went to the house. Constructing the outbuilding had to wait until the following year; I wanted the main house finished first, so I could move in sooner and stop paying rent for the house in Dolan.

20. The Inside Job

Once the house was closed in, we proceeded with the interior work. Much of the time it was just one contractor, who worked five hours a day, four days a week. The contractor was also the handyman for the area and he reserved the fifth day for fixing leaky faucets and other small jobs. This slower pace was much less taxing on me.

I continued to visit the construction site daily to discuss the project and get a list of what the contractor needed. When he needed something by the next day, I continued on to the supply stores.

Most of the materials were now small enough that I could transport them in the trunk of my car. Larger purchases, such as drywall, insulation and tile, were delivered by truck. One time a delivery of clay from New Mexico came on a big truck I had to meet in a parking lot in Snowflake.

I did a lot of driving that summer. The rough roads were so hard on the tires that I wore out a new set in about a year.

I sometimes had to spend more time inside the building supply stores, as it took time to find all the little items we now needed, and it took time to decide which commode or sink to buy out of the many choices. My respirator worked well, but it was not perfect. There was enough leakage so the insides of the mask smelled like the store after a couple of months, though I could just wash it off.

I discovered that I could last two hours inside the supply store if I ate two donuts right before I went in. Raising the blood sugar level can sometimes be used as an MCS remedy. This became a bad habit, together with the fast food I ate on my trips to town. It was simply not possible to both manage the project and keep up the perfect diet.

Construction trash accumulated around the work site. I hauled it away myself to the dump on the way to Show Low, when I had to bring my trailer along anyway. This saved me the cost of renting a dumpster.

The money kept rolling out of my wallet, but no longer at the dizzying speed it did while framing the house. The financial "housing bubble" started to burst that summer, when a lot of banks folded. That happened to my bank in October, but the FDIC stepped in and transferred my account to another bank without any loss. The new bank did not issue checks, so I had to transfer the account to a local bank. The local bank gave me immediate access to my money, allowing me to continue construction without interruption.

I considered using steel studs for the interior walls. They are more inert than wood, but it is a lot of extra work to wash off the manufacturing oils. My adviser did not use any steel studs in her house and the contractor didn't like working with them, so we did the interior with wooden studs, too. We used Douglas fir and hem fir (western hemlock), as available, with the bottom plate of rot-resistant redwood.

I wanted steel doors throughout the house. The only models available were for exterior use, with foam insulation, but they worked fine inside as well. They came with a glued-together door frame of pine that a local door shop replaced with less-odorous poplar. I never painted the steel doors or the frames. All the doors were 36 inches (90 cm) wide so I could use a wheelchair if I ever had to.

I had wooden blocks installed in the bathroom walls that were used to mount grab bars by the toilet, shower and sink.

I wanted the house to be usable in my old age, since moving to any sort of assisted living would be impossible.

The electrical wiring was installed in the walls using regular ROMEX cables. I made sure to get a brand without the coating that made it easier to pull them through conduits. This precaution may not have been necessary, as they were later encased in the walls of the house, and all ROMEX cables contain plastic and flame retardants anyway. My adviser had used a brand of ROMEX with the coating. She just wiped them with paper towels, and it worked fine for her.

My contractor twisted the ROMEX cables with a power drill before he installed them. The cable was simply mounted in the chuck as if it were a drill bit, then the drill was run at a very slow speed. Twisted wires reduce the magnetic radiation by about 90% (but doesn't reduce the electric field). Some brands of "12/3" ROMEX cables happen to be twisted already. These were used by my adviser, who just didn't use the extra "red" wire. I saved a little money by not buying these cables.

It is possible to further reduce the fields radiating from the household wiring by encasing them in steel conduits, but that was expensive and not needed in this house since I was using low-voltage DC electricity and not much of it. The only cables I enclosed in steel conduit were the feeder to the breaker box and one cable going to an outlet I might one day use for some electronics.

The house was wired for both 12 volt DC and 110 volt AC electricity. The DC wires were a little thicker, but otherwise there was no difference at this stage, and the inspector made no comment. He was curious about the twisting of the wires, but had no objections.

We used plastic wall boxes for the switches and electrical outlets. (Steel wall boxes can create stray currents on walls covered with foil if one is not careful. Some inspectors also require the use of steel conduit when using steel wall boxes.) We sealed around the ROMEX cables entering each wall box, so fumes from the walls could not enter the wall box and drift into the living space. Insulation foam in a spray can works very well for this.

The 110 volt AC breaker box was placed on the outside wall. It was mounted on the steel siding, but with a spacer so there is no electrical contact with the siding. This removes one common path of stray currents.

Our building code did not require the grounding of metal siding and we didn't.

I was optimistic enough that we put "twisted pair" computer network cables in the walls. It's cheap to do before the walls are closed, and much harder later on.

Next was the plumbing in the walls. As I mentioned earlier, I decided not to use PEX, even though it is cheaper than copper. The contractor asked if I wanted him to solder the pipes together the standard way, or to double the amount of solder to be absolutely sure there was never a leak. I chose "double," even though it cost more labor time. The solder was lead-free, of course.

It took a lot of time soldering all the small copper pieces together for all the necessary bends. I constantly had to go to town to pick up just a few extra ¾ inch 90° elbows, ¾-to-½ inch adapters and other small pieces. It was slow going.

The drain pipes were regular hard ABS plastic. The only thing unusual there was that the contractor combined the three vent stacks before going up through the roof. The vent stacks prevent air from getting trapped in the drain pipes, allowing the effluent to move along unrestricted. Having just one stack going through the roof reduced the risk for roof leaks later on.

With the plumbing and electric completed (called rough-ins), it was time to put insulation in the exterior walls. We used formaldehyde-free fiberglass batts, which arrived with stinky asphalt-coated kraft paper on one side. We tore off the kraft papers and discarded them. They were intended to be the vapor barrier, but we later added our own when the walls were sealed.

The fiberglass insulation still stunk, but not terribly so, and I trusted that the seals we later put on would work, as they did.

When it was time to order the drywall sheets, I went to each of the four vendors in the area and bought a sample sheet of each brand they had in each store. Some stores carried the same brand, but I still got samples from every batch.

I returned home with about six samples. I cut a large piece off each sheet and put it in a cleaned one-liter glass jar, screwed the lid on and put it out in the sun. After roasting in the sun for an hour or two, I carefully sniffed each jar. The next morning, I ordered a truckload from the least odorous batch. As each batch can be different, I could not do this test earlier.

The delivery truck that came with the drywall and insulation was too big to make it up my driveway, but the driver used a little forklift attached to the truck to make the delivery. They were a different brand of drywall than I had ordered, so I sent them back.

The salesperson in the store told me she had personally instructed the workers in the warehouse which pile to take my drywall sheets from, but they still loaded the wrong kind.

They had also forgotten to include three sheets of fireproof drywall, to use in the closet on the side of the house.

The truck returned the next day with the correct sheets.

The drywall was used as the walls and ceilings in most of the house. In the bathroom, and all around the windows, we used cement boards, as those areas can get wet from condensation. Instead of smelling like insulation, the house now smelled of fresh drywall.

The drywall was mounted so the bottom was about an inch (25 mm) above the concrete floor. When the floor tiles were installed, the drywall was still higher than the floor. This was a mold prevention feature in case there was ever a spill, as the drywall would not wick up the water (this feature has already saved two houses from flood damage). The gap was later covered by a tile baseboard.

The seams between the drywall sheets were taped with regular paper tape and then covered with a less-toxic joint compound called Murco M-100.

Then it was time to seal all the drywall. This had three functions: a vapor barrier to prevent condensation in the outer walls, a shield against radiation from future cell towers, and a seal to block fumes from the wall materials.

Many regularly built houses have a vapor barrier. It is usually placed between the drywall and the insulation, using a variety of materials, some of which are not very tight. We placed the barrier on the room side of the drywall, and made it airtight to block fumes from the drywall, insulation, wood terpenes and plastic wiring.

Without a vapor barrier, humid inside air can migrate through the wall and when it is cold outside the water vapors will condense inside the wall and make the insulation wet. Wet insulation is a mold hazard, which is why many building codes in America require a vapor barrier (including our local code). The same goes for ceilings below an unheated attic.

It is a mold hazard to seal walls this way on houses in hot and humid climates, such as East Texas and Florida. Here the moist outside air can migrate inwards through the walls and condense, when the house is cooled with air conditioning. In such a climate the vapor barrier must be between the insulation and the siding, or not installed at all, as specified by the local building code.

The question is what to do in a climate like Northeastern United States, where the summers are hot and humid, and the winters are cold. I wish I knew.

There cannot be two vapor barriers in an exterior wall or attic ceiling, as water might get trapped. A storm with high winds and heavy rain may drive water inside walls that are normally dry — then those walls must be able to quickly dry again. As the house ages, there may also be small leaks.

The insulation we used (formaldehyde-free fiberglass without kraft paper) allows water to pass, but some insulation materials act as a barrier.

I have seen several houses in Arizona that have sealed walls like mine. Some are twenty years old, so it seems to work very well in our dry climate.

I know one house in the hot and humid climate of East Texas, where the walls were sealed. During a later renovation they found a lot of moldy insulation inside the walls.

Some building inspectors may be uncomfortable with sealed walls, simply because they have not seen it before. We avoided any such problems since the inspector never saw it, but I know of houses where the inspector saw it and approved.

We used aluminum foil to seal the walls and ceilings. It was put on like wallpaper, but with no overlap between the foil strips. The glue cannot dry when trapped between two aluminum sheets, so a gap of about an inch or so was always left between the strips of aluminum. This gap was later covered with aluminum tape.

We used "heavy duty" aluminum foil from the grocery store, as well as 3 ft (1 m) wide rolls of 1 mil (0.025 mm) aluminum foil from the Alufoil company. It won't work to use stiffer foils, such as Denny foil, which will quickly get loose. I got the aluminum tape from E.L. Foust in Chicago, that sells a tape with a glue I (and my adviser) tolerated the best. Even though most of the glue is covered by the tape, enough fumes can escape to be a problem when using a lot of the product — we used about twenty rolls for the whole house. The tape and foil were installed using a smoothing tool for wallpaper (a plastic ice scraper works too).

We used regular wheatpaste wallpaper glue. Some people have had problems with blistering foil, but they mixed the powder in cold water and didn't follow the instructions on the package. It is also best to throw away the bottom dregs of the wheat paste. We had no problems at all, and it all looks good ten years later.

The manufacturer of the wheat paste we used has since added a mold-retardant to the product. Make sure to check the contents or make it from scratch.

It is possible that the foil could become energized if there is an accidental electrical short. This could happen if a nail were driven into the wall and accidentally damaged an electrical wire inside the wall. Building inspectors may require that foil is connected to the ground wires for that reason. Some people have simply connected their foil to the ground at every electrical outlet by using aluminum tape and grounded steel outlet boxes. This often works, but could backfire if there is a lot of dirty electricity or the ground wires actually carry a voltage (which they often do). I didn't ground my foil as there was no need, since my house used low voltage electricity. If I were to use regular 110 volt electricity in my house, I would probably do the same and just live with the tiny risk, as several other people do. Otherwise I might ground the foil at a single central location in the house (to avoid stray currents) and have a dedicated grounding wire go directly from there out to the ground rod under the electrical panel. There are now special grounding kits available for shielding paints that should work well with the foil.

Another option is to install GFCI breakers for all electrical circuits. These are called Residual Current Devices in some countries. However, some models generate a lot of high-frequency dirty electricity.

With the walls all foiled, then the bottoms of the walls were sealed to the concrete floor with aluminum tape. The gaps between the drywall and the wall penetrations (i.e. electric wall boxes) were also covered with aluminum tape. Water pipes passing through the walls were sealed with caulk.

The shiny aluminum walls were washed down to remove any oxides and oils, so the paint could adhere well. We used a TSP (trisodium phosphate) type detergent, but other kinds may work as well.

The taped seams were then puttied to make a seamless surface. The M-100 joint compound can work, though we used a homemade kind, using a friend's secret recipe.

The walls were painted with the same homemade clay paint my adviser used. The recipe was invented by a friend who kindly let us use it on the condition that we did not share it with others. It was all-natural ingredients, most of which I got from a clay store in New Mexico. The contractor then mixed it in buckets on site.

This paint had no preservatives in it, so it may work well only in a house with low humidity inside. I would use it only in a desert environment in a house without a swamp cooler.

Five of my neighbors didn't paint the foil on their walls, but left it as-is. It takes some time to get used to. Others have used the M-100 product as "paint" on their foil. There are also recipes for natural clay paints on the web, but make sure to test for tolerance and how well they adhere to foil.

I spent a lot of time deciding which floor tiles to buy. They come in many colors and widely varying prices. I bought various samples to look at, and several samples of the final two choices. My final choice was a special truckload offer, but when I went to buy them, the whole load had just been sold to the four rental houses that the state of Arizona was building for people with EI. I got another design, which I actually liked better.

We used tiles in many places: all the floors, the walls and ceiling in the bathroom, in the shower, around doors and windows, as baseboards, on the counters and as backsplashes to protect the clay paint in the kitchen.

We had to make our own thinset and grout, since all the commercial mixes have various added chemicals that make them faster and easier to work with. I have smelled the difference between houses with additive-free and commercial mixes. There is a difference, even a couple of years later. To me, it was worth it to pay the extra cost of labor.

Additive-free thinset and grout have been used to mount tiles and mosaics for two thousand years, but it is more labor-intensive than using the modern mixes. The contractor must be skilled and patient to do it well, or the tile will later get loose. The surfaces and the tile had to be thoroughly wet before setting the tile, and they must be wet-cured. The tile must be set on a very firm surface, such as cement boards, otherwise a degreased lath is needed. The tiles for the walls and ceilings had to be individually "buttered" on the backside before setting them and then the contractor had to hold each in place for a few seconds before letting go.

Someone in my area has since improved on the method to make it faster. He primed the cement board walls with lightly diluted "white glue" (Elmer's Glue/polyvinyl acetate, PVA), which was left to fully cure for some days. Then the thinset could be troweled on the wall for about 6 sq. ft (0.7 m²) at a time, with no "buttering" of the tile. The tiles could also be repositioned. This all saved a lot of labor.

To make our own grout and thinset, we needed about 600 pounds (300 kg) of super-fine sand, such as "120 grit sand" or "marble dust." It was not available locally. I visited a gravel pit, where they told me they sometimes produced some very fine sand for a golf course, but the sample they gave me was coarser than the 60 grit sand I could buy in bags from a local hardware store.

The only vendor I could find was a masonry supply store in Phoenix. I contacted two trucking companies, but they wanted $500 to $700 to bring the bags up here. Then I made a deal with a supply store in Flagstaff, that regularly got supplies from Phoenix and sometimes delivered to our area. This dramatically lowered the transportation cost.

I knew someone who was also building an MCS house at the time. She reported trouble with loose tiles, though I think she didn't use an experienced tile setter. To be sure, I asked my contractor to put some test tiles on the wall in the bathroom. He did, while varying the moisture level of the thinset. He knew in advance which was best, and he proved it to me. That tile had to be chiseled off, while he pulled the others off with his hands. None of the tiles he installed have fallen off.

The cabinets for the kitchen and bathroom were of steel with a baked-on powder coated paint. They came without counter tops, which we made ourselves using cement boards with 18 inch (450 mm) floor tiles on top. It looked beautiful and has held up very well.

We didn't use any recessed ceiling lights, as they are difficult to seal. We just used regular ceiling dome lights mounted over electrical boxes. The insulation on the back of the dome lights was discarded. Doing this is probably against the building code, but I didn't want hot fiberglass insulation in my airspace. Without the insulation the lights may run too hot with the 100 watt bulb they were rated for, but I never intended to do that anyway.

The project was moving along nicely, but it was getting late in the year.

21. The Last Winter in Dolan

I expected the weather to become too cold for camping around the start of November, when I had to return to Dolan Springs for the winter, but it was an unusually mild fall that year. We had light frost most nights from the start of November, but I was well-equipped with a good sleeping bag, and the days were still warm.

I knew my time was limited and made sure to buy all the important materials the contractor needed for the winter, such as tiles, cabinets, light fixtures, sinks, faucets and ingredients for the paint.

Three days after Thanksgiving the temperature dropped to 14°F (-10°C), which is the coldest I have ever slept outside. My sleeping bag was rated for 20°F (-7°C) and with the outer bag it was supposedly okay for -20°F (-30°C), but those ratings are always quite optimistic and I was so cold I had to stay awake and stir in the bag for hours late at night.

The following day it slowly warmed up into the forties (about 7°C) and a chilly wind blew from the north. There were only five days left in November, but I was waiting for a delayed shipment of steel kitchen cabinets from Chicago. I had to inspect them upon arrival to make sure they were not dented, so I stayed on. Two days later the weather warmed up again, but it was no longer stable.

Since it was now the Christmas season, I bought a string of solar-powered lights to hang on a juniper bush near my tent. The LED lights were bluish-white and nobody in the neighborhood could stand to look at them, so I threw them out. They bugged us even at a great distance. It could not be

EMF, it had to be the light itself, but how? I didn't tell this to any outsiders, as that would just be another reason to think we were all crazy. Nine years later, in 2016, I read an article in the magazine *IEEE Spectrum* about how the new bluish-white LED street lights bothered a lot of people and interfered with nocturnal animals. It wasn't just us after all.

A winter storm was approaching a week into December when I finally had to high-tail it back to Dolan. I felt well enough that I was able to make the drive in a single day.

We had now been working on the house for more than five months, but there was still a lot of work to do. With most contractors I would have stopped for the winter and resumed construction the next spring, but I was fortunate to have such a dependable contractor that I could leave while he did the painting, tiling, cabinets and fixtures on his own. I kept in weekly contact with him over the phone, where we discussed the project and he told me how many hours he had worked, so I could send him a check. He had almost all the materials he needed, but a few times I had to go select an item at the Home Depot store in Kingman, so he knew what to buy at his local store.

I asked the contractor to be at the house by 9 a.m. on the shortest day of the year to see how far the house cast a shadow towards where the solar panels would be mounted. I had calculated the distance, but I needed to be sure that the panels were not shaded by the house during the winter.

I was surprised that I felt better inside the Dolan house during my last winter there. I could stay inside more without getting brainfog, I could use the heating system while inside and I did not have problems tolerating my car. Being away for about six months seemed to have desensitized me, just as I had gotten desensitized to foods by not eating them for a long time. Perhaps owning two or three homes and rotating residence every few months can work, just as rotating foods helps keep food allergies at bay? Of course, that method requires a lot of money.

The heating system was not yet installed in my new house, but it was super insulated and designed to let the winter sun help heat up the house through the big south-facing windows. How much that helped was apparent when it got really cold in January. When the contractor arrived one morning, it was 8°F (-13°C) outside, while a thermometer sitting on a north-facing window sill showed 42°F (6°C) in this coldest spot in the house. As the sun shone through the windows, the house warmed up some more. That's pretty good for a house with no heater inside yet.

A storm dumped a lot of snow on Snowflake in early February and the road to the building site was not plowed. First it was covered with snow and then it became muddy once the snow melted, so the contractor didn't make it out there for a week. A few weeks later he got the flu and lost another week of work.

The most time-consuming work was all the tile. There was a lot of tile in this house. The floor was the easy part, while it was slower to do the walls and ceilings in the bathroom. Even slower was the tile around the doors, windows, baseboards, and the backsplashes in the kitchen where they needed a lathe to adhere to.

This was my fifth winter sleeping on the porch in Dolan. My neighbor to the north seemed to burn more firewood than the other winters, creating a problem once the wind shifted from his direction in February. Many nights I was awakened by the smoke and had to sleep with a dust mask on. By March my lungs hurt much of the time and I had herniated a muscle from all the coughing, but then it started to warm up again.

The news that I was soon vacating the house in Dolan travelled widely and I was contacted by multiple people who were interested in renting it. In March a woman and her son drove from California to try it out for a night, but she decided to stay where she was.

The contractor told me in April that he was finished with the interior, so I drove over there to inspect my house. He washed the floor and moved all equipment outside the house, to let me test how well I felt inside. I felt fine. There was a dusty smell from the clay-painted walls, but that was all. I was very pleased.

The mid-April weather was cold and windy, so I stayed just two nights before driving back to Dolan.

Back in Dolan I focused on packing and getting ready to move. When I called the electrical company to cancel their service, the woman asked if I was moving out of their service territory. I replied that I was moving beyond any service territory and would make all my electricity myself. She thought that was very cool.

I was concerned about bringing any mold spores from the Dolan house. I therefore made sure to store all books and papers in plastic tubs. I also washed all my clothes in borax and gave them a lot of sunlight on the clothesline.

I did not have a lot of things and packing took just a few days. I was eager to move.

22. Moving In

I moved in ten days after my inspection visit. My friend, Nevada-Jack, transported my belongings with his truck and cargo trailer and returned to Dolan the next day.

It was now late April and spring was in full swing. It was 34°F (1°C) the first morning, warming up to 70°F (21°C) in the afternoon, before plummeting to 40°F (5°C) the next morning. The temperature fluctuates dramatically in the dry, thin air of the high desert. The heating system was not installed yet, and it was just 50°F (10°C) inside the house the first morning. The house wasn't quite odor-free yet, so I slept outside in my tent. I was confident the house would offgas over the summer.

The house had a slight odor of vinegar, from some caulking the contractor did a few days before, but he had used aquarium caulk and the smell lasted for just a few days. The medicine cabinet in the bathroom was made of glass and steel, but it had a few stinky plastic strips. I had to remove the cabinet door and leave it in the shed for a few months. The house otherwise just smelled dusty from the clay paint, which was now six weeks old. I kept the windows open all day and closed at night to air out the house and warm it up. The lumber in the walls also needed to dry — even kiln-dried lumber contains a lot of water.

There was no heat, electricity or running water in the house yet. That would come later.

I carried water in a bucket from the outdoor faucet to flush the toilet, wash the dishes, clean, etc. Water for cooking and drinking came from a vending machine in town, where I filled my five one-gallon (3.8 liter) glass bottles. I did my laundry in a bucket with a washing-plunger, while showering took place at a friend's house. (I later learned when visiting someone who was building a house that it works well to shower by kneeling in the bathtub while pouring water over me with a big mug. The water came from a two-gallon (8 liter) steel bucket placed inside the tub. The water was heated on the stove and then tempered by adding cold water.)

I used flashlights the first couple of nights, but then I had a small, temporary solar electric system rigged up to feed electricity to the house wiring. It was able to power only one of the ceiling lights at a time, but that was all I really needed.

I cooked on an outdoor propane camp stove, just as I had done in Dolan, and I still do today. The stove sits right outside the kitchen door where it is sheltered from the wind and this setup works well, except for a few days a year when the weather is terrible.

I used two coolers with ice to store food, until I got a refrigerator. My new propane refrigerator was delivered a week after I moved in. The trucker did not want to drive on dirt roads, so I had to meet him out by the highway with a helper and a flatbed trailer. The propane fridge was very heavy. It took three men to lift it.

I could not have any propane inside the house, so the fridge sat on my covered porch, where it was fueled by a portable propane tank. This worked well, except when the wind blew out the little pilot light. The fridge was moved inside a small utility closet on the side of the house, when it was ready a couple of months later.

Life was getting organized and fairly comfortable. Most important of all was that I felt better than I had for years, as long as I didn't go anywhere.

I felt well in the house with the windows open, and it got better over the summer. I slept inside for the first time one stormy night a month after I moved in. I was a bit groggy in the morning, so I continued to sleep outside, except during bad weather. I could probably have slept fine in the tiled bathroom, but I was so used to sleeping outside that it didn't occur to me.

The place was amazingly quiet. Sometimes I could hear the wing beats of a single bird and the rumble of a train nearly twenty miles (30 km) away.

I arrived with very little furniture: just a patio table, some wooden folding chairs and my old steel hospital bed. A friend gave me another patio table. Patio furniture of glass and steel is commonly used in MCS homes, as most regular furniture is too toxic.

I bought several chrome wire-shelving units, which do not gather dust and work very well. I also bought a large steel-and-glass patio table, but the paint on it was a problem, even after it had sat outside for three years. That is the only piece of patio furniture I have ever had such problems with.

The road to my house had now been registered with the county for a year, but it was still not on the various GPS navigators and map websites. That took another couple of years. It took five years before the county installed a street sign.

I made sure detailed driving instructions were placed on the first package I had delivered. The UPS driver followed the instructions and had no trouble finding his way. He then entered the information into their internal database where later drivers could look it up.

The other delivery service, Fed Ex, gave me trouble for years. The driver was somehow unable to remember where to go, even after coming out there multiple times. Packages were returned "undeliverable" or re-routed to people they somehow knew I was friends with. I had to tell vendors not to use this service. The problems disappeared when a new driver took over the route.

Getting regular mail service was not difficult. A month before I moved in, I had the contractor install a mailbox at a convenient spot along the mail route — eight miles from my house. A few days after the registration form was handed in, mail started to arrive in the new box.

It still took several months before all the mail order companies received the new address from the Postal Service, so their computers stopped complaining that my address was invalid when I called to place an order.

There was no trash service available; I had to store my household trash, and then haul it on my trailer to the dump every couple of months. I had to do it every four weeks in the summer, because the heat made the trash stink. I always combined a trash run with a shopping trip. It was not much of an effort and cost a lot less than using a trash service.

There was no telephone service in the area. When I called the local phone company the year before, they refused to discuss extending their lines before my house was built. Once when I saw one of their maintenance people, I stopped and asked about it. He said they typically charged one or two thousand dollars a mile. That seemed reasonable since I needed the lines extended two or three miles, depending on how they routed it.

Now that I was living there, I called the phone company again. They sent someone out to look and then they said it would cost more than twenty thousand dollars. I complained, and then they said they might do it for fifteen thousand. They normally did it cheaper, but they deemed my area as slow-growth, so it would take too long before they would get more customers on the new cable.

I had no telephone the first two years. I had a separate line at a friend's house, which gave me voice mail that I picked up a couple of times a week. That worked fairly well, but most people in our modern hyper-connected world would probably find it quite unacceptable.

My brother eventually built a sort of remote controlled cellular phone, where the transmitter and other electronics were placed far from the house. Inside the house I had a simple traditional phone. This worked well, though it was a complicated project to build and install, and not something easily duplicated.

Some cell phone companies have since started offering fixed wireless devices to entice people to give up their landline (and kill off the competition). Ordinary landline phones are plugged into this wireless device, instead of the usual plug in the wall, and works just like on a landline (except when the wireless reception is poor, of course.)

I know a man with severe EHS who installed one of these devices a hundred yards from his house. It is connected to the house with a twisted pair (Cat 5e) cable encased in a buried steel conduit, and with a line filter. This all serves to reduce the microwaves travelling along the cable.

23. Finishing the House

The contractor took two weeks off to take care of some other projects shortly after I moved in. I used the time to get organized for the summer's projects and to haul several trailer loads of construction trash to the dump. I was also able to return $350 worth of surplus materials.

The contractor had other jobs to take care of that summer and worked fewer hours each week. By August he started on another house and could only work for me one day a week. There were also a few delivery problems with materials arriving much later than expected.

The slow pace suited me fine, as long as we could essentially finish before winter. I wanted to stretch out the expenses and since I no longer paid any rent, I had more money available each month. Since I didn't have to visit the supply stores so often, I also felt much better and could enjoy whole days with very few symptoms.

The main project for the summer was to build an outbuilding to house the solar system and all the machinery that made noise and EMF, i.e. the washing machine and the two pumps. One pump circulated the hot water for the radiant floor, the other took low-pressure water from the storage tank and sent it to a pressure tank so water could flow fast out of the faucets and shower nozzle. Higher pressure was also necessary for the reverse-osmosis water filter I later installed.

I originally planned for a larger outbuilding with a small guest toilet, but with money so tight we built it smaller and without the bathroom. We made it 10 x 14 ft (3 x 4.5 m), which was just small enough that the county inspectors did not have to be involved. This saved me both fees and hassle, as well as paying property taxes on the structure.

We broke ground for the outbuilding in late May. The backhoe also dug the hole for the pole for the solar panels and made the trenches for the gas line and other buried pipes. The yard looked like a moonscape. The wind blew hard the next day with loose dirt flying everywhere, forcing the contractor to give up and go home for the day.

We lost a couple of weeks to various delays, but by mid-June the foundation was in place and the water pipes connected up to the house. The booster pump could first be installed when the outbuilding was closed in, but for now I had gravity-fed water for the faucets and toilet. Showering had to wait until there was full pressure on the pipes.

It was difficult to find a propane company that would deliver to my address, as I was further out than any of their routes. The company that delivered to a neighbor two miles away did not accept new customers.

One company said they would extend their route if I could find them another customer in my area. Fortunately, a married couple were building a house a mile away while living in their motor home. They were tired of hauling their own propane and were glad to sign up. The company then came out to install a big propane tank and the underground gas lines.

I bought a propane generator to run my well pump and washing machine once a week. I wanted a big enough generator that could also run a clothes dryer if I had to buy one (I never did), so I bought a 7500 watt model. It weighed 340 lbs. (170 kg) and sat on a concrete pad with a direct line to the big propane tank. Propane is much cleaner than gasoline and I never had to haul any fuel myself. A 5000 watt generator would have been plenty, but I didn't know that at the time. The vendor offered a twelve-month no-interest account, which helped stretch out my expenses.

The generator was designed for use in huge RVs and runs much quieter than most generators, which can be extremely noisy.

By the end of July, the outbuilding was framed, so the booster pump could be set up temporarily. A week later, the utility closet on the side of the house was ready. It was sealed off from the house, allowing me to have propane appliances there without fumes entering the house. The propane refrigerator was installed right inside a door from the porch. The propane water heaters for showering and the heating system were installed behind another door to the same closet. Steel pans were installed under the water heaters to protect my house against mold damage in case one of the heaters ever leaked. I was now able to take hot showers.

I tried to drink the well water a month after the line was connected to the house. I first used a filter where the water slowly trickled from an upper reservoir through a carbon filter, using only gravity flow. I got a stomach ache every time I drank the water, even though the lab test showed the water to be safe.

Once I had more pressure on the water, I had a reverse-osmosis filter installed. This worked – now I could drink as much of my well water as I wanted and no longer had to haul water from town in glass bottles.

The in-floor radiant heating system was then hooked up. Embedded in the concrete floor were four loops of PEX tubing which were now hooked up to a non-electric manifold. The manifold had four valves that I used to adjust how much of the hot water would go to each of the four loops.

A PEX tube then went through an insulated trench over to the outbuilding where the circulation pump was located. From there the water went back to the closet on the side of the house where the propane water heater warmed it up again before returning to the manifold. This way the heating system was totally noise-less and non-electric in the house.

The outbuilding also had a PEX loop embedded in the concrete slab. In the middle of the winter I could turn a manual valve to direct the warm water through the loop to keep the outbuilding frost free. I never intended to keep the outbuilding at room temperature, so the slab is not as insulated as the house (it's a monopour with insulation foam underneath and along the outer perimeter instead of a stem wall).

This has all worked very well. The water is about 95°F (35°C) when it enters the floor of the house. It is about 75°F (24°C) when it comes back from the floor and continues on to the outbuilding. Houses that are not so well insulated may need to use higher temperatures (and accept higher heat loss).

One day some cattle transporters dropped about a hundred free-range cows off near my house. I woke up one morning at 4 a.m. with a cow stomping and bellowing on my porch. Cows can damage a house by rubbing up against it, so I had to get gates and a fence erected around the house. That was an $800 expense I had hoped to delay until another year.

The last work done that year was installing the solar system, the circulation pump and washing machine, together with their plumbing and wiring in the outbuilding. I deferred some of the plumbing, wiring and drywall work in the outbuilding until the following summer to stretch my expenses.

By late October, the project was essentially completed and I called for the final inspection. The inspector I had made sure to get for each inspection had left for another job and a new inspector showed up instead. He lived in an off-grid house he had built himself, and he could see it was all put together neatly. No problem.

I knew one of the things they looked for at the final inspection was a full kitchen (in addition to running water, flushing toilet, lights, etc.). Since I cooked outside, I did not have an indoor stove. To take care of that, I bought a used electric stove as a prop. It was a nice model with a glass top I could use as counter space. I got it cheap as it had been hit by lightning and didn't work. There was a 240 volt outlet for the stove and I could argue that I could power it with the generator. The inspector looked at the stove, then looked sideways at me and just noted that I cooked outside.

The entire inspection took ten minutes, then I was issued an occupancy permit. Some jurisdictions do not allow people to live in a house before it is completed, but that was not a problem here.

The inspector reeked of cologne, but I had a powerful fan exhausting air out through a window and the house did not get contaminated. I know one person who refused to have the final inspection to avoid contamination and they eventually just mailed the certificate to her.

In early October I closed up the house and turned on the heat for the winter. I was now sleeping inside in a well-heated space with lights, running hot and cold water, a washing machine and air that didn't make me dizzy. After nearly ten years of living in places that didn't really work for me, I was finally in a house that really did.

24. Shielding

Microwave radiation from cell phone towers and other wireless sources has grown exponentially across the globe for the past two decades, and it will continue to rise for some time. Wireless services are now available in many remote areas and even national parks where visitors demand full access to the Internet. Public funds subsidize the installation of towers in lightly populated areas to bring wireless Internet to people who otherwise would not have access.

When my house was built in 2007, the contractor had to walk up a nearby hill or climb on the roof to use his cell phone. Five new towers have since been built within 20 miles (32 km) of my house, though not closer than about 10 miles. Today, cell phones have good reception anywhere in my yard and it is even possible to use the Internet wirelessly. I do not expect the towers to get close, since I live in an area without electrical service. The towers use a lot of electricity and it is expensive to build them off the grid with large battery banks and a backup generator.

Rural towers tend to be taller and have more powerful transmitters than those in the cities, since they cover a larger area. The ambient microwave radiation has risen more than tenfold since I moved here, though it is still fairly low and does not seem to be a problem for me.

In 2015 I travelled to Dallas and measured the ambient levels there to be about 10,000 times higher than at home.

When building a healthy house today it is prudent to consider installing shielding, especially if building in a populated area. It is much easier to shield a house while it is being built than to do a retrofit.

Shielding is done by wrapping a room or a whole house in shielding material. This is called a Faraday cage. Like any cage, it is essential that there are no holes for the radiation to pass through, just as a sturdy lion's cage is worthless if the door is left open. This means that to make a basic shield, it has to include all the walls, ceilings, doors and windows. The floor may also need shielding.

Most modern building materials do not prevent cell phone signals from entering a house. This includes gypsum wall boards, plywood, plastic siding, cement boards, tar shingles and plain glass.

There are two types of shielding materials: absorptive and reflective. The absorptive materials absorb some of the radiation as it passes through. The thicker the material, the more it absorbs. The absorbed radiation is turned into heat, though the absorber won't get noticeably warmer.

Examples of absorptive materials include bricks, concrete, clay, wood and special carbon-based materials. The drawback to this type of shielding is that very thick walls are required to provide meaningful shielding.

Reflective shields are easier to work with. They work by reflecting the microwaves like a mirror, using various metals such as steel, aluminum, copper and silver. The thickness of the material is not important, since even household aluminum foil can provide at least a thousandfold (99.9%, 30 dB) reduction of the microwaves.

The drawback to reflective shielding is that it reflects both ways: waves from the outside are reflected back out, and waves generated inside a shield will bounce back inside. This means that if people try to use a cordless phone or Wi-Fi inside a shielded room, their exposure will be much higher than if they stood outside with it. People may also be more affected when using computers and other electronics inside a shielded area.

My house has simple reflective shielding. This includes the steel siding, the steel roof and the steel door. The foundation has an eight inch (20 cm) thick stem wall of solid concrete, with aluminized foam board insulation on the inside and below the slab.

The aluminum foil sealing my walls and ceilings is also the second layer of shielding. Having two layers greatly improves the shielding effect, since the two layers can cover each other's weak areas, such as slits where plates are joined and holes where electrical boxes come through.

The windows have aluminum frames and low-E glass, which has a very thin metallic coating. Manufacturers are developing low-E glass that is not shielding, to allow cell phone signals to better penetrate office buildings, so specifying low-E glass may not be sufficient in the future.

There are three large windows in my house that are not low-E. They are on the south side to gather free heat from the winter sun. If I cover these windows with aluminum foil (such as aluminized "bubble wrap" like Reflectix) that side of my house provides about a hundredfold (99%, 20 dB) reduction of the cell tower radiation. When the south windows are uncovered, they provide no reduction at all.

A cell phone that had a decent signal outside the house ("three bars") reported a minimal signal inside the house with covered windows (alternating between "zero bars" and "no service").

If I need the shielding in the future, I could replace the plain glass with the metalized low-E glass or build a mesh-screen to cover the south windows. In both cases I would lose a lot of free solar heat in the winter, though it would be less with low-E glass that has a high Solar Heat Gain Coefficient.

Be aware that aluminum foil is also a vapor barrier, which can create condensation and mold if used in exterior walls and ceilings in climates where they need to breathe (ask a local building professional). This problem can be avoided by using copper mesh shielding or perforated aluminum foil. Perforated foil is sold as reflective heat-shields for attics, but is too thick to be used as wallpaper. Regular foil can be perforated manually with a tool called a "woodpecker." I have not experimented with perforated foil, though the tiny holes should not weaken the shield much in today's environment.

There are shielding paints available. I have not tried any of them, but they are very expensive and I'm told they are also very toxic.

The big question is how much shielding is needed. Is a factor of ten, a hundred, a thousand or even more needed? The human body appears to be affected by EMF logarithmically, which means that a doubling of the radiation level is probably not noticeable and even a ten-fold increase may not be terribly important. This is similar to our perception of light and sound, which is also logarithmic.

If a nearby cell tower or the neighbor's Wi-Fi or wireless smart meter is causing symptoms, a tenfold (90%, 10 dB) reduction is unlikely to be sufficient for relief. A hundredfold (99%, 20 dB) reduction may not even be enough.

It is not too difficult to build a house that provides a hundredfold reduction of microwaves. Higher levels are possible, but are much more involved and would probably require the help of a specialist, such as an EMC engineer. An alternative is to use multiple Faraday cages inside each other, such as a shielded bed canopy inside a shielded room inside a shielded house. If that much shielding is needed, it may turn the house into a prison. It may make more sense to relocate to a low-radiation area and use less shielding.

My house is shielded against microwave radiation from cell towers, Wi-Fi, cordless phones, etc. There are other kinds of EMF, which my house does not shield well against. They are more difficult to shield and I hope they will never be an issue in my area.

Frequencies higher than 6 gigahertz are presently used for microwave links, satellites and some radars. In the future they will also be used for portable wireless gadgets that communicate over short distances in cities, and possibly also directly to satellites. With these higher frequencies the wavelengths are so short it will be very difficult to ensure the inevitable holes and slits in a house shield are small enough. Perforated shielding becomes increasingly ineffective at higher frequencies and may become obsolete within a decade.

Lower frequency EMFs are also difficult to shield because they are better at penetrating the shielding materials. The lower the frequency, the more difficult it is to block, just as base sound waves travel through walls and ear protectors more easily than higher tones.

The shielding of my house barely affects the reception of radio stations (FM, AM).

For even lower frequency radiation, such as from electrical motors and wires, there are two kinds of radiation: electrical and magnetic. Neither is an issue in my house because I use 12 volt DC electricity and mostly for incandescent lighting.

If I used regular 110 volt AC electricity then the foiled walls would shield the electrical field from the wiring inside the walls. Aluminum foil does not shield magnetic radiation, which is why the wires were twisted. The twisting reduces the magnetic radiation about tenfold (90%, 10 dB), while further reduction would require covering the wiring with steel conduit.

It is not realistic to shield a house against low frequency radiation from the outside, such as from a nearby power line.

This chapter is a basic introduction to shielding with a focus on the simple shielding of my house. This is a complicated subject that may seem new and mysterious, but shielding has been used for decades at military and intelligence facilities and by military contractors to protect against surveillance and electronic weapons. They use sophisticated methods, materials and equipment to reach much higher levels of shielding than that used in my house.

25. Financing

I spent the rest of my savings battling the illness and for basic living expenses while I lived in the camp in Texas. When I was awarded a disability pension, I was given a lump sum for the time back to when I applied. This back pay, and what little I saved while living in Dolan, was enough to buy the land. Then I needed to finance the construction of the house. I've never had a mortgage, so this was all new to me.

I had two long conversations with a friendly loan officer from a large bank. She told me how a bank looks at loan applications. They consider income, credit history, savings and other factors to see how big a loan they think you can carry.

The bank also wants to be sure they can easily sell the house to cover their loan, if the owner cannot make the payments. This requirement is difficult to meet with an EI house, as it costs more than a normal house of the same size and may look unusual.

The general real estate market does not put a premium value on environmentally safe houses and a bank is probably not interested in the small specialty market for people with environmental illness. In their eyes, a healthy house costs more to build, but is not worth more.

A bank may accept the extra cost of tiled floors, as tiles are attractive, but other costly materials may not add to the property value. They will only loan out as much as they think they can sell the house for, so they may require the owner to put in more cash than for a conventional house.

A bank doesn't like houses they think are hard to sell. This means it has to look "normal." Shiny aluminum walls and other unusual features are frowned upon, though you could consider not telling the bank about them. It is also hard to sell a house that is a lot smaller than other houses in the area, or one that has just one bedroom. A local bank may be more flexible on these things than a big national bank.

Most banks also think a house that is powered by the sun and not connected to the electrical grid is too hard to sell, though I have since learned that some local banks in areas with many solar houses may issue such loans.

Another barrier is any deed restrictions (also called covenants). I have a friend who wanted to buy a house that had several deed restrictions, including one that only people with MCS could live in the house. This restriction was put in place when the land was sold off by the neighbor. The bank refused to issue the loan as long as that restriction was in place. Fortunately, they were able to get it removed.

Banks also want to protect their investment by requiring the use of expensive building contractors, which meant I had to pay more for the house. I'm told that in some areas the banks may also require that the soil under the house is soaked with pesticides to deter termites.

It was clear that a bank loan was not practical. There were too many problems.

I have since heard about government programs to provide housing loans to people with disabilities on a low income. I probably didn't qualify anyway and these loans can be more restrictive than a bank loan. However, the loan officer has more flexibility in accepting unusual features, if they are needed because of a disability.

My parents sent me $15,000 as a gift, but that was far from enough to build a whole house. It might be enough to build the primitive Remote Basic setup, but that was not feasible with the harsh winters in Snowflake, and I really wanted something more comfortable.

I asked around to see how other people had financed their homes. Most had financed their houses through their family in some form or another. One woman had half the money she needed and used low-interest "teaser" credit cards for the rest. When her house was finished, she got a mortgage and used it to pay off the credit cards. It is easier to get a mortgage on a finished house than a construction loan, as there is less risk for the bank.

I have a friend who slowly built his house while camping in his car and using a travel trailer, he didn't tolerate well. He financed the house from the money he saved by not paying rent plus his wife's modest income. After seven years he was able to sleep in the house, but he is still working on the house three years after he moved in. This was in a warmer climate where year-round camping was feasible.

My parents knew about all these considerations and offered to put a mortgage on their house and loan me the money. They had lived in their house for many years, so it was all paid off, and with their stellar credit rating they got the loan on great terms. Without my parents' help, this project would have been much more difficult.

The financing I now had was still modest. I needed to keep the costs down in many ways to allow me to buy the expensive healthy materials.

It was a huge cost savings to buy land that was four hours by car from any big city and two hours from any large town. Land that is well beyond commuting range is a lot cheaper.

The financial downside of such a location is that I sometimes had to pay extra transportation costs for building materials.

I saved money by building a modest-sized one-bedroom house of 800 square feet (80 m²). That is considered small in America, where the average new house is around 2400 sq. ft (250 m²). Being just one person, I had no need for a large house. On the other hand, it does not seem to me that much is saved with an even smaller house. The cost of installing a well, plumbing and electricity will not really be reduced further, as there still has to be one bathroom and one kitchen. The cost for the foundation and the shell of the house will not be reduced proportionally with the size of the house, once it's already a basic small house. Most of the environmental houses in Snowflake are in the 800-1000 sq. ft (80-100 m²) range.

I know of a tiny MCS house in Canada. It is built on wheels and has 160 square feet (17 m²) of living space. It cost $60,000 to build. That makes financial sense only because it is parked in someone's back yard with no expenses for buying land, well, sewage, etc.

Modern construction methods have evolved the way they have simply because of cost. Building a house that is as close to conventional construction as possible seems to be the most cost effective. Sealing the walls allowed me to use drywall and fiberglass insulation instead of costlier exotic materials. Natural building methods, such as rammed earth, adobe and straw bale, are very labor intensive and therefore costly unless you can do the work yourself (make sure you know what you are getting into).

Not having a bank loan also saved me a lot of money. A bank imposes various costly demands on a building project, to limit their risk. I was free to be my own general contractor, my own architect and to use any contractor. I think that reduced the overall cost by at least twenty percent.

The general contractor organizes the entire project, such as ordering materials, hiring and scheduling contractors, dealing with the building inspectors and overseeing all aspects of the project. An experienced general contractor can make a project go faster and smoother, as he anticipates the needs of the project so materials and contractors arrive on time. He can also prevent costly mistakes and put together a good budget.

I knew people who had been their own general contractor and done it well. With their advice, by hiring dependable contractors and working at a reduced pace, I was able to manage the project myself as owner-builder.

Managing a building project is not for everyone. It takes organizational skills, levelheadedness, ability to make decisions, ability to work with people, some technical understanding of the process and the stamina to show up at the worksite daily.

Some people have had a hard time managing their project, resulting in expensive mistakes, contractors walking off the job, big cost overruns, long delays and all sorts of problems. The personal impact can also be substantial. One person had to stop the project after a year to take a year off to recover before resuming. Another reported it took her two years to recover after her house was finished.

I didn't use an architect, either. It was not difficult to put together the drawings for a simple house, especially since I could borrow the plans for other houses to use as a template. I thoroughly enjoyed drawing up the plans for the house myself.

Another cost-saving measure was that I hauled a lot of the materials myself. My adviser had to hire someone to pick up all the materials at the building supply stores. Some contractors insist on buying their own materials, both to prevent mistakes and also to earn extra money from the markup, which can be very steep.

Shopping around for the materials saved me a lot of money. The prices of tile varied dramatically and one electrical supply house was willing to give me a contractor's discount and sell me electrical cables at a price much lower than the big-chain supply store.

I didn't rent a dumpster for the construction trash, but simply let it pile up on the ground. When I needed to haul materials on my trailer, I took some trash to the dump on the way to the store.

I didn't need to rent a portable toilet as that was not customary and the contractors did not expect one.

I made a loose budget based on what people told me the various phases had cost them, but it is hard to make a solid budget for a custom house.

There was a building boom in both the United States and China at the time, with shortages of raw materials and building products. This made the cost of copper wires, copper pipes, concrete blocks and other materials jump. I once saw a box of nails double in price within three months and when I ordered the steel panels for the roof, they cost $2000 — a year before that $2000 would have paid for both the roof and the siding.

The foundation cost a lot more because of the floor heating system. It was a surprise how much more than a simple "monopour" foundation, which was the most common type in the neighborhood.

There were also totally unforeseen expenses, such as $1000 for renting a water trailer and $3000 for fence work.

In the end, the project cost 20% more than my loose estimate. That is actually good for a custom-built MCS house managed by an inexperienced owner-builder. I have seen projects where the final cost was more than 50% above reasonable estimates. The more unusual a project is, the more difficult it is to estimate the cost. This is even a problem for professionals who have suffered cost overruns on some stadiums and other iconic buildings.

When the house was largely finished, I could see I did not have money to build the outbuilding. The outbuilding could not be delayed, as it housed essential parts of the solar and water systems. I reduced the cost by omitting the bathroom, making the building smaller and delaying some work until a year later, but I was still short nearly $10,000. I asked a bank if I could get a home-equity line of credit on the almost-finished house, which they agreed to, until they sent out an appraiser who reported that the house was not connected to the grid.

The appraiser just did a drive-by evaluation and didn't see the inside of the house, so features such as the tile work were not included in the appraisal. The appraisal was simply based on what the house looked like from the outside, its size and location, and what similarly-sized houses in the area had recently been sold for. The appraiser valued the house at a third of the actual cost!

I was glad that the bank turned me down, as I found a much better solution to finance the outbuilding. I used a "teaser" credit card and credit accounts from two building supply stores. They were all interest-free the first twelve months — after that it would have been the usual usury. I delayed paying my parents back and within a year I had paid off the two store cards. The teaser credit card was transferred to a new teaser card, which I then paid off on time. I could do it that fast, since I no longer had any rent to pay.

I never paid any fees, as I "transferred" to the second credit card by using it for all purchases the last two months before the first card expired, and used the savings to pay off the first card. The only interest I paid was a 1½% "introductory rate" on the new credit card.

This method was much cheaper than a bank loan, but I had to be very careful not to fall into any of the traps that would have resulted in fees.

An example of these traps was that one card was not always zero-interest — some purchases would accrue regular interest if not paid off within 30 days. And any payments on the card balance would only be applied to the high interest part once the entire zero-interest balance was paid off. This was hidden in the fine print, which I luckily read.

Credit cards should only be used at the end of a building project, and only by someone who will read all the fine print and who is organized enough to avoid the costly fees.

Some people have started on their house, expecting the project to take the three months it may take for a professionally managed cookie-cutter project in a big city. The EI houses in Snowflake typically took a year to build. A few were finished a little faster — some took much longer. It can be costly to arrange financing that depends on the project being finished quickly.

In my case, the house interior was finished ten months after we started. I then moved in and no longer had to pay rent while essentially camping in my house for some months. I stretched my expenses by working at a leisurely pace for the next six months to build the outbuilding and install the systems for water, electricity and heat. This all helped me finance the last part of the project.

I could have saved about $5000 if I had ended my lease in Dolan when we began construction. I lived in a tent in Snowflake for the first six months anyway, but then I spent five months in Dolan over the following winter. I could have spent the winter on a campground in the low desert near Tucson, but it would not have been pleasant.

If I had the concrete floor tinted, buffed and glazed instead of tiled, I could have saved about $1500. I didn't know anybody who had tried it, and the glazing has to be reapplied after some years, so I didn't try it.

I saved about $20,000 by building my home miles from the electrical grid. The price of land drops dramatically once it is a few miles from utility service and at the time the local utility charged about $12,000 to connect a new house on a large lot. The same utility has since changed its policies, and now pays some of the cost of connecting a new customer.

I had to pay about $4000 for my solar system and $3500 for a propane generator, which I use weekly to pump water and run the washing machine. The State of Arizona and the federal government gave me about $1500 as a subsidy for the solar system. My solar system is modest, but does everything I need it to. The cost of a solar system can range from a tiny RV-sized system for about $500 and up to a fancy system suitable for a solar sultan, that may cost $30,000.

People with electrical sensitivities may be affected by the typical modern solar electric systems, which use inverters, MPPT "optimizers" and pulsing charge controllers. Those problems can be overcome by good design and choice of equipment.

There must be at least a hundred off-grid solar houses in my area and seven of the EI homes are now off the grid. Living off the grid is a change in lifestyle and requires the owner to understand and interact with the system. It is not for everyone.

I could have saved $10,000 by not drilling a well and instead have water delivered to a tank by a truck. This is commonly done in rural Arizona, where wells often need to be 300-800 ft (100-250 m) deep. Most of the EI households in Dolan were on waterhaul, and the bank I talked to said they would finance a house without a well.

I estimate it cost about $2500 to super-insulate the attic and the walls of the house. That was a good investment, both in terms of saved heating expenses and increased comfort both summer and winter.

A commonly asked question is what it cost to build a truly MCS safe house. That depends a lot on how big the house is, the price of the land, what materials are used, the cost of the contractors, whether you manage the project yourself and how well you do it. These are all very important factors.

The typical Snowflake house is about 800 to 1000 square feet (80-100 m²), with one bedroom, one bath, well, grid electricity, and on a 20 acre (8 ha) lot. If built in the Snowflake EI neighborhood, using the "Snowflake method," using the same contractors and the project is managed well, the 2010 cost was around $175,000. Some people have spent less, some much more. The cost of building the same house in another area could be much higher. I do not have enough data to really know what the typical cost is for the other construction methods, though if they are more labor intensive they seem to cost more.

Many people have spent their savings on expensive treatments and expensive temporary housing. Be careful about running out of money — make sure there is enough left for a down payment on a house.

26. Home Safe Home

It is now eleven years since I moved into my house and sixteen since I left Texas. When I lived in the camp outside Dallas, we sometimes talked about Arizona and New Mexico as the Promised Land: go to the desert, breathe the clean air, live without EMF and you will be healed. Reality wasn't quite as simple, but I have never regretted that I moved out here.

It is a joy to live in a house that is comfortable and safe with very few neighbors. The indoor air quality is exceptionally good. Most gaussmeters and radio-frequency meters show nothing inside the house. I enjoy the expansive views of the desert and seeing the Milky Way stretching across the dark night sky. There is less wildlife here than in wetter climates, but the desert is far from dead. I see roadrunners, ravens and groups of antelope meander through. Packs of coyotes can often be heard howling in the distance. I do not miss the flying insects.

Since my home is heated and powered by the sun, I maintain a sense of connection with the outdoor weather and the daily and annual cycles.

My home is rather sparse compared to many houses in the United States, since even almost-inert materials are a problem if there are a lot of them (as I found out the hard way). I use mostly steel-and-glass patio furniture and keep my house rather uncluttered.

The warm soft tones of the desert are reflected in the colors on my walls and floors. On my walls hang glass-enclosed pictures from my travels and a friend's painting of a coyote howling at the moon. I have seen many creative ways people have decorated their homes without bringing in unhealthy materials. It is important to feel comfortable in our homes to see the full health benefits from them. I like my home, and I like that it takes good care of me in many ways.

Giving my body a safe and restful place to live was not a cure. My sensitivities to chemicals, pollen, mold, light and electromagnetic radiation did not disappear, but I have a much better quality of life and I have become more resilient. When I fill up my car, I no longer need to take the elaborate precautions I described in the start of my first book. Today I simply use a disposable glove, hold my breath while setting up the hose and stand upwind from all fumes, though I sometimes still need to use a respirator. It may not seem like an improvement that it now takes about fifteen minutes before my mind gets foggy in our local Safeway grocery store (thus I still shop with a respirator), but such a cushion allows me to "act normal" in places I could not before.

I had to hire someone to type this book from my handwritten manuscript. I still cannot use a computer in a meaningful way, but I am now rarely affected by brief encounters, such as with cash registers in a store or walking past someone talking on a cell phone. It helps that people do texting more now, instead of yakking on their cell phones while waiting in the checkout line. I place the shopping cart to give me the most distance to any electronic gadget, while it still looks "natural" to any outsider.

I go shopping once a week. I wear my respirator, though the stores make my clothes smell, so I still get affected when I take the respirator off. When I get home and take a shower, I recover pretty well. I have two sets of outer clothing, one for going to town and one for around the neighborhood. Once or twice a year I go to some sort of outdoor event, such as a

Native American dance festival, a parade or a street fair. I do not wear the respirator and just accept the effects. It may take a couple of days to recover, but sometimes I just want to play "normal." I do not want to pull up the drawbridge to my safe castle and fully shut out the world. People have done that and their safe haven sometimes turned into a prison that was very hard to get out of again.

I know that these modest gains can quickly be lost if I moved to a less-safe house or had to stay in a hospital.

I operate my home with various air quality zones. The safest zone is the house itself, where I rarely allow anything new until it has spent time offgassing in the other zones.

Some things are left outdoors initially. This includes any boxes I receive, which I open on the porch. Books, magazines, photocopies and mail go to the outbuilding for offgassing. Groceries go to the refrigerator or sit in the vented closet with the refrigerator until they are ready for my pantry. More toxic items are kept in the garden shed. This is all organized so well it is easier than evaluating each item to see whether it needs offgassing or not. I still need to read using a reading box, glass plates, sheet protectors or a respirator.

When I first came to Dr. William Rea's clinic in Dallas in 1999, he tested my blood for twenty common chemicals. I had up to 29 times more of some of the chemicals in my blood than the average American.

Dr. Rea did a new test in 2010, using new technology that checked for hundreds of chemicals at a fraction of the cost. This time all the numbers came out well below the averages. Very few chemicals were even detectable. Someone else from my community did the same test with similar result. Our safe housing and lifestyle obviously make a difference. Sadly, Dr. Rea passed away in 2018.

The safe house has allowed me to solve a puzzling issue: I had noticed that I got symptoms from radios, fans and refrigerators — even at a great distance. Even my Swedish tube-telephone gave me symptoms after a while. It didn't make sense that the radiation from those weak sources should reach that far.

I experimented by sitting eight feet (2.5 m) from a battery-powered radio with the sound totally off. That did not affect me within ten minutes, but when I turned the sound on it was a problem. When I put on heavy-duty ear protectors, so I couldn't hear the radio, I was fine again. I realized that the sound itself gave me the same type of symptoms that I get from EMF and sunlight, such as the burning sensations. This makes some sense since all three are frequency waves. I also discovered that distorted sounds, such as from telephones and low-quality radios, were worse than less distorted sounds. Clear sounds, such as human speech and even violent weather, did not produce any symptoms. This may explain why some people have a problem talking to callers who use a cell phone — the microwaves cannot possibly travel through the phone system, but the sound quality is generally lower than landline phones.

I'm affected by any kind of recorded music, even music I've loved for decades and still love today, but have no problem with live acoustical instruments.

It seems that my trouble tolerating the low-EMF car was mostly the sound of the noisy engine. I still have problems if I have been exposed to too much EMF/light/sound, but then it helps to wear heavy-duty ear protectors while driving. I still use a modified diesel car.

I have since found other sensitive people with the same problem. Their coping methods include watching movies on low-EMF DVD players with the sound turned far down and subtitles turned on. One uses heavy-duty ear protectors when she travels on an airplane.

I have lived in four different time zones with very different climates and vegetation. Each time I made a major move, I felt better for a few years, simply because I was not allergic to the local pollen, terpenes and mold. We have those in the rural Southwest, though generally less than in wetter climates.

The first time I visited the Southwest was on a vacation in 1991. I noticed that my nose wasn't stuffed up, as it was back in Ohio. As my allergies got worse, I asked an allergist whether I should relocate to a desert city, such as Phoenix or Albuquerque. He replied that he didn't think it was helpful any longer since so many people had moved there and brought along non-native plants, some of which pollinate profusely in the new climate. The result was that the big desert cities have seen some of the highest pollen counts in the nation, though Tucson and Albuquerque have since banned some of these plants.

When I moved to Dallas from Ohio, it took just one year for me to become allergic to the local vegetation, and it quickly became a problem most of the year. I didn't get allergic to the vegetation in Dolan Springs, though some people there did. Perhaps I didn't live there long enough, since it took five years before I was affected by spring pollen in Snowflake.

People with severe food allergies often rotate their foods to manage their allergies. The same can be done with houses and a few people actually do that. If I had enough money, I might have a winter-spring house in Dolan Springs and a summer-fall house in Snowflake.

All parts of the desert have a lot of very fine dust in the air. It can easily be seen on a dark night with a powerful flashlight pointed upwards. This dust is a problem for some people.

Every year there are forest fires and prescribed burns in the region. The smoke plumes can travel for hundreds of miles and reach most parts of the Southwest. Every year there are days when I keep the house closed up because I can smell smoke from these fires.

The desert sun is fierce, especially for those of us who are light sensitive. I cope by using wide-brimmed hats, special long-sleeved sun-protection clothing, very dark sunglasses and occasionally a non-toxic titanium sunscreen. I mostly hike at dawn and dusk, but sometimes I get overexposed and have to cover the windows and stay inside for a couple of days.

There is no perfect place on Earth. Some people feel better by the ocean or in the forest or even in a city. We all just have to find out what works best for each of us.

I hope this book has given an idea what it entails to have a house built. It is not a task I recommend for everyone. I have seen projects get into all sorts of trouble and some that never succeeded. I even know someone who committed suicide when she couldn't live in her new house.

Make sure the person in charge is up to the task, that he or she has the skills, stamina and personality that are necessary. Also make sure that the goal of a house you can live in is not crowded out by secondary goals, such as what it looks like or the view from it or to use the latest cool "green" materials.

I firmly believe that my house turned out so well because I followed a proven method I knew worked for me. I knew that because I visited a recently finished house I felt good in, and I copied the methods and materials. I had seen too many "safe" houses I could not live in and I did not wish to gamble.

I had to pioneer a few things with the heating and electrical systems, simply because I had nobody I could copy, but with regards to how the house was constructed, I followed good advice.

The method I used is not the only one that reliably works, but I think it was the best one for my situation, including finances, climate, time frame, abilities and level of sensitivity.

In the first years in my new house I was visited by someone who spent a night and told me she really felt good in my house. She wanted to build one just like it except she wanted to do everything different!

Building a house can be an amazingly creative experience, as it was for me. Many environmentally sensitive people are very creative and many are also non-conformists — including myself. But, it can be hazardous to be a non-conformist MCS builder. Of course, experimentation is what has taught us what works and what doesn't, but be careful! There are many ideas floating around and some are presented with much enthusiasm, even though they are not really well tested, or haven't even worked well. People have run into trouble by trusting that the latest "super-duper-eco" or "formaldehyde-free" material actually worked for them.

Before I moved here, I had many days with brain fog so bad that I forgot what I had just read when I got to the bottom of a page. It is hard to study up on safe building methods for many of us, but relying on verbal rumors and postings on social media can cause a lot of trouble. Building a safe house is an enormous expense. Few of us can afford to gamble with that much money.

Some methods do not work in all climates. Using preservative-free clay paints or unfired adobe in a humid climate is probably a mold hazard.

Sealing the walls with airtight aluminum foil, as I did, is a mold hazard in warm and humid climates, such as Florida and East Texas. This is because when the humid air enters the wall from the outside and is cooled down by the house air conditioner, water can condense in the insulation and make it wet. In such climates the wall needs to breathe or be sealed on the outside of the insulation, neither of which can be done correctly with a tight seal on the inside.

Sealing the walls has been used successfully on several houses in northern Arizona, but I'm not certain about other climates. Ask a local building professional.

The contents of building products sometimes change, often without any change to their labels. An example is the wheat paste we used to attach the foil to the drywall. A few years later, the manufacturer added anti-fungals to the formulation. Someone using it to put foil on her walls got sick from it; when she checked the Materials Safety Data Sheet (MSDS) she discovered the change. She had to pull the foil down again and start over.

I have also heard about shipments of magnesium oxide sheets and ceramic floor tiles that were contaminated.

Another issue is that people's sensitivities to building materials vary. I know of people who live happily in houses with large surfaces covered with wood. That would not work for me, even if it was less-aromatic wood such as poplar or maple and it had offgassed for years. I have no problem with additive-free concrete, but some people are strongly affected. Even the Snowflake houses are not universally tolerable. The bottom line is that there is no method and no set of materials that is guaranteed to work for everybody.

There are several green building certification programs. The scientist Anne Steinemann published an article in 2017 where she looked at such programs in several countries. She found that many of these programs allow a building to receive their highest ranking without addressing indoor air quality at all. These programs cannot be used as a guideline whether a house is healthy to live in or not.

All the planning, testing, checking and good advice paid off with a house that was successful for me. Most MCS houses I can't live in very well, but this one worked for me and most visitors seem to like it, too.

My house has worked out well in other ways. The 12 volt DC solar system has worked without failure — unlike the local grid which has outages every year.

The heating system has also worked well and reliably. The inside temperature is comfortable almost year-round, even though I have no air conditioner and the temperature is above 90 degrees (32ºC) most summer days. The heavy floor and the extra insulation act as a thermal flywheel that evens out the day/night temperature, which in our thin and dry air can swing 40 degrees (20ºC). I just need to keep the windows open at night to cool down the house. (This won't work in Arizona's low desert, where it does not cool down enough at night.)

In the winter the house is so comfortable I walk barefoot on the heated floor. I really like that there is no noise, no blowing air, no fumes and no EMF. It was even comfortable when we had a serious cold spell down to 20 below (-30ºC). The double insulation and the passive solar heating save so much propane that the gas company once called to ask why I use less than their other customers.

The only thing that has broken so far is the kitchen faucet. It started leaking into the cabinet underneath. Fortunately, I discovered it in time and now have a zero-EMF water alarm and a glass tray below the sink. Some EI houses have no cabinets below their sinks to make leaks visible right away.

I didn't intend building more fencing than just around the house, but I had to add some more over the years. The free-range cattle tore up the land with their hooves while using my property as a beeline for their daily migrations. I also needed to deter humans from entering my property from the back side, including a hunter who used my hill as a lookout for deer, and two guys who came in on all-terrain vehicles at 2 a.m. with the obvious intent of breaking into my house (they ran off when I turned on the porch light).

A great benefit of living in the boondocks, well beyond the electrical grid, is that there is very little development. Most regular folks are intimidated by dirt roads and having to be their own electrical utility. It is easy to spot outsiders as they drive slowly on the dirt roads in their shiny, spotless vehicles, and they do not wave like the locals do. I hope the county never paves the roads and that the electrical grid stays away forever.

A drawback to living in the country is that developers like to place objectionable projects there. People in the country tend to be less likely to mount effective opposition to a project, and developers usually have little trouble convincing the local politicians to support their plans, even what may not be in the best interest of the host community.

Northeastern Arizona hosts four coal-fired power plants that make electricity for cities hundreds of miles away. These plants are some of the most polluting in the nation and three of them waste copious amounts of precious ground water with their cooling towers.

But developers were surprised by the resistance they ran into when there were plans for building a nuclear power plant in the early 1990s. The project was cancelled after fierce local opposition.

The year after my house was finished, a neighbor discovered that an enormous wind farm was planned for our area. It would place giant wind turbines next door to my house.

Four people from our EI community went to visit an existing wind farm to learn more about them. One woman had seizures just looking at the turning blades, a phenomenon called photosensitive epilepsy. (We later found a scientific article about how it can be caused by wind turbines.) The same woman also gets seizures from strobe lights, which is common among epileptics.

I seemed to sense the infrasound half a mile (800 m) downwind from the turbines (a phenomenon described in Dr. Nina Pierpont's book *Wind Turbine Syndrome*). Then there were other potential problems, such as new power lines, ground currents, noise, etc. It was clear that there was a real danger that I could be forced out of my new home.

It is common that developers try to keep quiet about their plans as long as possible to give the neighbors very little time to organize protests, or even find out before the bulldozers arrive and it is too late to protest. The official notifications to us neighbors arrived just a few days before the planning and zoning hearing, but fortunately someone found a website promoting the project to investors, so we had a two-month advance warning. Once the hearing date was set, a handful of us got organized and handed out flyers.

A hundred people showed up to protest at the hearing, the chairman said he had never seen so many people there. Two newspapers sent journalists to cover the hearing. One gave a detailed coverage of the project without mentioning the protests at all. The other paper focused on the protests.

Other developers had plans for wind farms in the general area and three grassroots organizations sprung up to oppose some of the projects. It took eighteen months, but then the controversial projects were dead and the county had a new ordinance in place that offered the residents some protections and required the developers to be open about their plans well in advance.

It was interesting to watch the political process. Politicians can be called upon to make decisions on a wide range of issues and it is impossible for them to be well versed in everything. Here they struggled with unfamiliar issues, such as noise levels, infrasound, strobe lights and how far a loose turbine blade could fly.

It was hard to be part of the opposition. People were nice to hold some of the strategy meetings outside so I could participate, but the hearings were in a meeting hall I could not be inside for long. I had to wait outside until it was my turn to speak at the podium for the allotted three minutes.

Over the course of the campaign, I was several times so worn out I had to spend a day in bed in a darkened room to recuperate. I could not have participated without my safe house to support me. This illustrates one major reason why the environmental illnesses have still not been accepted, even though Dr. Theron Randolph published a book about MCS as early as 1962. We are simply too disabled to show up en masse in the halls of power, and we are too old to have outraged parents do it, like it happened for autism.

It was strange to oppose a project I liked in principle, but once green technologies become industrialized and run by money-people, they can become a lot less green. It is not in the spirit of "green" to try to rush through such a big project. That approach seemed to backfire as it upset a lot of people.

Green technologies are not always safe for people with environmental illnesses. I cannot drive an electric or hybrid car and I avoid post-consumer recycled paper because of the contaminants (such as from mold and carbonless copy paper). Green energy projects can also be problematic, since many of them generate dirty electricity from the inverters used in both solar and wind systems. Wind turbines also produce noise, flicker and infrasound that seem to trouble sensitive people more than regular folks.

The solar thermal plants use mirrors to generate steam to drive a turbine. This may seem safe enough, but it involves many tons of toxic oils to transfer the heat to the turbine building. In 2015 the *Arizona Republic* newspaper reported that the solar plant near Gila Bend had been leaking this chemical for several months with the neighbors complaining about a smell like burning plastic.

Every year environmentally sick people travel to the Southwest in the hope of better health. It can be a frustrating experience going from place to place and trying out houses that are safer-than-normal, but not safe enough — or houses that are great but not affordable.

Safe housing that is affordable is in very short supply and can move fast. A good strategy may be to accept living in a more marginal place and cope as well as possible, while looking for something better or having something built. The Seagoville camp and the house in Dolan Springs were such stepping stones for me, and each was better than the previous place. If I had waited until the perfect place became available, I might never have made it to Arizona.

The Snowflake community grew gradually, where people slowly bought land adjacent to each other, or started satellites in the area as I did. There is no master plan and no covenants protecting the neighborhood. There have been several attempts at creating planned EI communities by buying and subdividing tracts of land. Examples are the Escalante House project in Utah and an unnamed project near Hay Hollow outside Snowflake, but too few people signed on so they never happened. The only such project I know that actually happened was Quail Haven north of Tucson, but only two houses were built there, with a third built on a large nearby lot.

The Snowflake contact person, Susan Molloy, receives about a hundred phone calls each year from people looking for safe housing. I do not have data on how many actually settle in the Southwest, but the Snowflake community typically welcomes two newcomers each year. There would be more if it was easier and cheaper to settle here, but having to build or convert a house deters many people.

Most people with severe MCS or EHS live on a reduced income and cannot afford to buy or rent a healthy house. The state of Arizona built four reduced-rent rental houses for people with MCS or EHS who live on a low income, but the waiting list is very long. More affordable rentals are urgently needed. Too many people have to live in cars, vans, trucks, tents and trailers.

People usually hear about us by word of mouth or through social media, though one man didn't know where to go, so he called the Arizona governor's office and amazingly enough the staff there had the answer.

It takes some pioneering spirit to pack up and head West, though the EI communities have all kinds of people, including artists, engineers, police officers, car salesmen, college professors, nurses and more. We even have people from Canada, Europe, the Middle East and Asia.

Most of us used to live in big cities and many prefer to be near a large town. The largest EI communities are around Tucson, Prescott and Santa Fe, with their benefits and drawbacks compared to the rural communities.

I used to think that I could never live in a city smaller than a million people, but was surprised that I actually liked rural living, and not just because of the landscape, the night sky and the environmental benefits. I like the friendly and unhurried people that are so rare in the big cities. I have seen much kindness from strangers, such as the time my car broke down while driving through the hamlet of Woodruff. Within minutes, a man came out of his house to ask if I needed help. Twenty minutes later a retired mechanic was on the scene. Someone drove me to get the needed spare part and within a couple of hours I was on my way again.

I have only once seen graffiti in Snowflake. It was done with chalk!

I enjoy living in the Snowflake community where I can invite a group of people over, or go to someone's house, and not be concerned about people making me sick with fragrances, dryer sheets or wireless gadgets. That is very liberating.

Many of the town people are used to us and sometimes help when there is a difficult situation. One recent example was when a community member died and a memorial service was held outdoors so we could all attend. The service was to be held in the yard of a local church, but the road in front of the church was repaved the morning of the service so the pastor moved it to a local park.

I realized I had MCS in 1996, four years before my health crashed. I wonder what would have happened if I had found competent health care that early and moved to a healthy house in the desert right away. Would my health have stabilized so I could continue to work and live a normal life? I'll never know.

It was not easy to get to where I am today, but if I had to start over again, I would build the same house in the same place, with just minor design changes.

Afterword

A fair question that must come to many minds is: can people really be *that* sensitive? Even after all these years, I still get surprised.

While writing this book I went to visit a friend. I've always felt well in her house, which is built like my own, but this time I could smell fabric softener. I easily identified the culprit as a shirt hanging over a chair, out of several pieces of clothing that were draped over her chairs. We moved the shirt outside and the house was soon fine as usual.

It was then that my friend told me she had worn the offending shirt the previous day. She had been home all day but had gone outside to meet a visitor (we usually receive visitors outside). The visitor's clothes smelled strongly of fabric softener. Even though the two people had no physical contact and didn't stand closer than about six feet (2 m), enough of the fabric softener was absorbed by my friend's cotton shirt to stink up her living room.

Fabric softener is one of the things I am most sensitive to. Had it been something else it might not have been a problem with such a minute amount, just as it didn't offend my friend.

Recently I had another friend visit me in my home. After about fifteen minutes my sinuses started to burn and my mind was getting "foggy." To save money she buys used clothing at thrift stores and then washes and airs them for a long time to remove the chemical residues left by the prior owners. She was wearing such a recently broken in piece of clothing, which she hadn't told me about. Neither of us could smell anything, but I started recovering soon after I lent her some of my clothes (I keep a bin of guest clothes in various sizes).

I have had several of these experiences over the years with both chemicals and electronics. The worst is when the exposure is so low that I cannot detect anything so I stay exposed until the symptoms really hit. Then it can take days to recover.

I know two people with MCS who have no sense of smell at all. Not having this warning system greatly complicates living with MCS, but it also serves as proof that we're not just affected because we know it's there, as the skeptics like to postulate.

MCS and EHS are very complex diseases with a great variety of sensitivities, symptoms and timelines. It sometimes takes a very controlled environment to figure things out. My home and neighborhood can provide that, but for people who live in less optimal housing it is much more difficult and confusing. It is no wonder that some exposure tests fail to support the existence of MCS and EHS because the researchers clearly did not understand the complexities and failed to do their tests in a truly controlled environment. (These tests did not eliminate common triggers, such as fluorescent lights, ambient radiation, noise, ambient air pollution, dirty electricity, computers, etc. Some also didn't account for delayed reactions. Most also did not even screen their test subjects.) Despite their many shortcomings they continue to be touted as "proof" that environmental illnesses are purely psychological.

Allergies can be complex, too. Some people get mild discomfort during pollen season, some break out and have tears and a runny nose, yet others get inflamed sinuses and become dizzy. Some people get anaphylactic shock if they eat a single peanut.

In the second chapter of this book I told the story about a physician who said that allergies were a fad and that I definitely did not have allergies. Now, more than twenty years later, the story can serve as an important lesson. I doubt that there are doctors making such flippant remarks about allergies any longer, and one day that will also be the case with chemical and electrical sensitivities.

The February 2016 issue of *Scientific American* (p. 40) says that twenty percent of antibiotic prescriptions are for people with chronic sinus infections. Before I could control my environment, I had to take one round of antibiotics after the other for my sinuses. I wonder how many other people would not need antibiotics if the doctors instead suggested they and their families get off fragrances, fabric softeners, the so-called air fresheners and all the other unnecessary chemicals that pervade the lives of most people. Chemical exposures cannot cause sinus infections directly, but they may enable them by suppressing the immune system in the nasal tract so any bacteria or viruses that happen to be present suddenly have free reign. I have noticed the connection between chemical exposures and sinus infections many times myself. The above mechanism is my own speculation and it is not proven, but recently a similar mechanism was documented by Ellen Foxman at Yale University, who found that when people get chilled their immune system is less active, thus the reason for "catching a cold."

The government spends billions of dollars researching treatments for illnesses. Would it not make sense to research preventing illness more? The medical industry has no interest in losing business, and many special interests would rather their products were not proven a health hazard, so such research has to be publicly funded and be free of industry influence. We need answers to questions such as why has the rate of autism skyrocketed in just a few decades, and why do younger people get cancer much more than before. They cannot be explained away by better awareness, detection, or other explanations that are sometimes rather flippantly used.

Some people may think that if I could build my own house then I couldn't have been really sick. Why didn't I make a living building houses for others?

My house was an extraordinary effort that wasn't sustainable and not commercially feasible. I didn't do any of the work myself because I could not operate any power tools or be near many of the fresh materials, such as lumber, grout and insulation. Since I was in charge, I could control a lot of things that otherwise would be difficult or awkward — even small things such as turning off the generator and standing in a safe upwind spot when I met with the contractor.

I also had to keep the project moving slower than would be acceptable for a commercial project. These are just some of the barriers I faced and there would be more if I tried to make it a living. Despite giving myself more accommodations than would be realistic with a commercial project, there was still a health impact. I could tell the difference when I had multiple days off and I even had a period when I couldn't drive to the construction site. My effort was clearly not sustainable.

I have a few times seen people get up from their wheelchairs and walk around. Or someone elderly who psyched herself up to attend an important birthday with a smile on her face, even though it was hard. That doesn't mean they were faking it on a normal day. Sometimes people can temporarily go beyond their normal limits, but that is something able-bodied people cannot possibly understand.

The impact and difficulty of living with environmental illness is very difficult for outsiders to comprehend — even if they read this type of book carefully and multiple times — simply because it is far beyond the experience of most people. A book cannot really convey what it means to have a substantial disability to someone who is healthy. It is perhaps like trying to describe a glorious sunset to someone who was born blind. Unfortunately, there are many who have blinders on while they claim with great authority that they see and know everything.

Many people probably consider the science and practice of medicine a hundred years ago as rather primitive. It would not surprise me if a hundred years from now people will think the same about today's medical system. Despite all the advances, much about the human body is still not well understood. It is only within the last decade that gut flora (the gut microbiome) has become accepted as vital for human health and that the adult brain can regrow neurons. It was thought for decades that our genes were fixed, but now we know they can self-modify through epigenetics. In 2015 scientists at the University of Virginia discovered that the brain is directly connected to the immune system. Those are all major discoveries that refute long-standing medical dogma and there are surely many more textbook-altering discoveries to be made.

Various kinds of anesthesia have been used for well over a century, but nobody knows how they actually work!

Medical scanners can present us with dazzling pictures of our brains, but they can't show whether a person has a headache or not. There is still no way to objectively measure headaches and other forms of pain, or even a simple itch. We have all experienced these sensations so we accept that they exist, even though they still baffle medical science. Just because something cannot be measured by our current technologies doesn't mean it doesn't exist.

Unfortunately, that humbling insight is rarely applied to less universal symptoms, such as "brain fog," paresthesia and the other symptoms some of us experience when exposed to chemical or electromagnetic triggers. Without accepted objective diagnostics and with a disease that doesn't fit neatly into the current medical paradigm, we are often subjected to suspicion and dismissal by the very people we go to for help.

In the recent past physicians commonly believed that migraines, asthma, multiple sclerosis, fibromyalgia, Parkinson's, lupus, and many other diseases were due to "hysteria," "repressed emotions," or similar vague psychological labels. It was also once a commonly held belief that unaffectionate "refrigerator moms" were the cause of autism in their children — a cruel burden of blame to lay upon the mothers. Until recently physicians believed stomach ulcers were caused by stress, but now we know the culprit is the bacterium H. pylori.

When I was a child, I heard the adults talk about someone who was "afraid of cats and dogs." Allergy was not a household word in those days and to outsiders it did look like people were "afraid" of the animals they were allergic to.

It is a quite normal human response to be apprehensive if a big menacing guy approaches with a bullwhip in his hand. I don't think any reasonable person would contradict that statement, simply because we can all understand the situation. But if we substitute the menacing man with a situation that is equally threatening — but only to *some* people, while it is innocuous to others — then we tend to quickly reach for the psychological labels. This happens even to people who are highly respected, such as when former prime minister of Norway, Gro Harlem Brundtland, announced she had electrical hypersensitivity while she was head of the World Health Organization. Or the ex-First Lady of Germany, Hannelore Kohl, when it was made public she was extremely light sensitive.

The medical professionals are as guilty of that as anyone, especially when the issue is controversial. Physicians are generally expected to quickly reach a straight and orderly conclusion and are not used to prevaricate, or even discuss, a contentious issue. It is much safer and more convenient to throw the patient into the garbage can filled with psychological labels, most of which can't be objectively verified or repudiated.

Giving people a psychological label can have real consequences. It can mean that the patient's legitimate problems are ignored, with no further attempts at reaching the correct diagnosis and instead a focus on inappropriate treatments. Psychoactive medicines can have very unpleasant side effects and the patient can be pressured into taking them by misguided physicians, family members and disability insurance administrators.

There can also be a substantial impact from being stigmatized with a psychological label. The family, medical system and others will tend to not take the patient's needs seriously, especially requests for accommodations such as avoiding pesticides, fragrances and electronics. Being treated poorly by the medical system makes people trust it less and be more reluctant to seek medical assistance for any kind of need that is not an absolute emergency, as documented in a

2016 study by professor Pam Gibson of James Madison University. In some cases the system has gone amok and forcefully hospitalized people or removed their children, as chronicled in the book *Prostituting Science: the psychologisation of MCS, CFS and EHS for political gain,* by Diana Crumpler.

Accepting there is a legitimate disease is also necessary to get funding for scientists to study it and hopefully find out how to cure and prevent it, or at least further improve the acceptance.

In the early 1990s I was dating a schoolteacher. One day one of her young pupils was scratching himself a lot, so she sent the child home with a note asking the parents to check for lice. The irate mother called the school and said that *her child* couldn't possibly have lice. The child did have lice — I know that because my girlfriend got them and she gave them to me too. All too often the reaction to embarrassing news is to attack the messenger.

The existence of a group of people who are profoundly affected by a wide variety of common chemicals and electronics is not only embarrassing to some very powerful special interests, but a direct threat. That is a large and sordid subject that in many ways is unfolding like the tobacco wars and the asbestos controversy did, and not something I will try to cover here. There is a section of the bibliography at the end of this book that lists several books that will shed some light on the resistance to accepting environmental illnesses as legitimate. Most of the listed authors are affiliated with universities; nine of them are professors.

For a historical perspective on a previously contested illness, see *Asbestosis: Medical and Legal Aspects,* by Barry Castleman. The asbestos industry was able to delay the inevitable for many decades by manufacturing doubt upon the research and painting the sick people as mentally ill, just as it is done today.

Albert Einstein once remarked that politics is more difficult than physics. Eventually, a political balance has to be found between public health, civil rights and simple decency on one side, versus inertia, convenience, practicality, cost and basic greed.

It is very difficult for us to be heard in the halls of power as we get sick when going there to speak out. With the slow progress and the many obstacles yet to be overcome, it can be hard to believe in a future where people with environmental sensitivities have better access to safe housing, schools, transportation, public places, medical facilities and a life less on the edge of society. But then consider that if someone in 1970 said that in thirty years most Americans no longer smoked, and the remaining smokers had to go outside, people would have simply laughed.

I remember in 1994 when I sometimes went to a farmer's market and felt lucky if I returned with a single small organic bell pepper — which often featured a wormhole. The sale of organic foods has since exploded in response to consumer demand and is now a staple in many regular grocery stores.

These changes came gradually and they could only have happened because enough people changed their minds and their habits. If cigarettes were banned, it would not have worked. The ban would not have been accepted and people would have gotten their tobacco anyway. If smoking in public places was prohibited too early, people would just have ignored it. The crucial part was to let the laws follow the gradual acceptance by the general population.

Of course, such acceptance is difficult to obtain and was helped along by public health warnings, individual doctors counseling their patients, the availability of smoking cessation programs, the rising cost of tobacco and even insurance policies that cost more for smokers. Making smoking inconvenient by restricting where people can smoke may also have helped later on.

Creating today's abundance of organic foods didn't happen overnight either. Growing organic foods is not just a matter of stopping the spraying of pesticides on the crops; it took time to develop the growing methods and a program for certifying that foods are organic, etc. The early adopters of organic food were willing to pay high prices for produce that looked rather scrawny, but the high prices attracted more growers and the prices gradually came down. This all happened without encouragement from the government.

More people are questioning what is in our foods and the packaging around it. What is the baby bottle made of and does it leach into the milk? Why does our food contain these unpronounceable chemicals? What are the long-term consequences of genetically modifying our foods and allowing a corporation to gain a virtual monopoly?

Suddenly a tipping point is reached and what was considered avant-garde yesterday becomes broadly accepted where the politicians and manufacturers will have to follow the lead of the people.

Several major manufacturers of household cleaners and personal care products have quietly phased out some of the most toxic ingredients in their wares and manufacturers of electronics and furniture have reduced their use of flame retardants. One major brand of antihistamine has been available in a dye-free capsule for more than a decade already.

Wheelchair ramps were not generally available until a few decades ago, even though wheelchairs have been in use for at least a century. The ramps did not suddenly magically appear, but came about because disability activists kept demanding them and were eventually heard. One of the pivotal moments of that struggle was when a group of demonstrators left their wheelchairs and crawled up the hundred steps on the front of the U.S. Capitol in what became known as the "Capitol Crawl of 1990."

Sometimes the authorities do have to lead, once there has been a big enough outrage. The Environmental Protection Agency (EPA) was created in response to Rachel Carson's book *Silent Spring,* while the auto industry had to make their cars safer following Ralph Nader's *Unsafe At Any Speed.*

AIDS exploded in America in the 1980s and was a certain death sentence. The disease challenged much dogma about infectious diseases and had a multitude of symptoms that varied with the person. It was thus controversial, but it was hard to argue against dead bodies. The authorities thought it was a problem confined to the gay communities and ignored it for years, as chronicled in the book *And the Band Played On* by Randy Shilts. Today, AIDS can be managed with drugs and no longer means certain death.

MCS and EHS will create their own story toward acceptance, scientific understanding, treatments and accommodation, but it will not be easy. As environmentally sensitive people become more visible, there may be a backlash. This already happened in the early 1990s, after several newspapers wrote sympathetic stories and some large manufacturers were sued by workers who got sick working in their factories. The backlash included several tabloid-style TV programs that painted MCS as a psychiatric illness and the doctors treating us as quacks. There were even articles falsely accusing us of being "afraid" of technology and wanting to live like "hermits." I have met people who told me they were against any kind of accommodation for disabled people – even ramps and bathrooms for people in wheelchairs. They considered that "special treatment," and thought nobody should be treated "better than others." I have seen a compilation of hundreds of anonymous comments to a YouTube video about some of the people in Snowflake. Most of the comments were quite hostile.

I'm not aware of any specific hate crimes against us, but I was once threatened simply because I had MCS. The man didn't know me. He angrily said that if people with MCS didn't live here in Snowflake, there would be several factories with well-paying manufacturing jobs (very unlikely). He then ominously stated that he knew exactly where our neighborhood was and then angrily took off in his pickup truck. This was several years ago, and nothing actually happened, but it would be easy for people angry at environmental regulations and the decline of manufacturing jobs to use us as scapegoats.

We are still very far from having safe housing and safe medical facilities available to those who need them, but there is some progress.

People used to smoke anywhere they wished in a hospital, then it became restricted to waiting rooms and cafeteria, and now it is outside only.

Our local hospital in Show Low, Arizona, requests its staff not to use fragrances, and the program is successful. I have heard that some other hospitals have done the same. This happened after the local EI community met with the hospital management. I have not heard of any American hospitals trying to limit patient exposure to electropollution, but some Swedish hospitals do.

A local dentist has a non-toxic and low-EMF clinic that I feel totally safe in. I just schedule the appointment for a time when they do not run air conditioning or electric space heaters, though I know they've turned those off for other patients.

Of course, most medical facilities are still not accessible to people with environmental disabilities, including nursing homes, pharmacies, labs, dental clinics and doctor's offices. In the past couple of years, I've visited two that were so heavily fragranced that my respirator was of little help — one clinic burned scented candles all day, every day.

Besides banning fragrances of any kind, detoxing medical facilities also involves making better choices as to which types of gels, creams, sanitizers, cleaning agents and many other products they use. Better ventilation is often needed as well. Creating a lower-EMF medical facility is much more difficult, since wireless equipment is so pervasive. Many hospitals rent out space for wireless transmitters on their roofs, and inside wireless computers, wireless patient monitors and other electronic equipment is everywhere. Many clinics now require new patients to enter their information directly into a wireless tablet computer and no longer have any paper forms. Sometimes electronics are built right into the hospital bed and wireless sensors attached directly to the patient.

Housing for people with environmental sensitivities has become better, but there is a long way yet to go. According to an old-timer, about 80% of the attempts to build a safe house failed during the 1980s. The success rate is much better today, though I still see new houses the owner can't live in.

The cost is higher than a regular house and often out of reach of the people who need it the most, since they are too sick to work and have to subsist on Social Security or other assistance. There are a few housing projects in Canada, Switzerland and the United States, where the rent is subsidized to make it affordable, but the need far outstrips the supply.

Far too many people live in housing that is marginally workable, at best, since that is all they can find and afford. Many are also terribly lonely since their friends and family are unwilling to limit their toxic lifestyle. It is no wonder some of us migrate to areas with EI communities.

The protests against the wireless smart meters was the first large campaign to limit people's exposure to electropollution. When these meters came to Arizona, I estimated the number of people who'd want to opt out to be in the hundreds — maybe a thousand. The largest utility in Arizona, APS, reported in 2014 that out of a million customers, no less than 19,000 opted out!

The Swedish professor of neuroscience at Lund University, Leif Salford, has called use of mobile phones "the world's largest biological experiment." Time will tell whether they will earn their place in the public mind together with Agent Orange, DDT, cigarettes, asbestos, leaded gasoline, PCB, hexavalent chromium, thalidomide, Love Canal, Fukushima, Bhopal, the Flint water system, the man-made earthquakes in Oklahoma, the toxic cloud from the burning World Trade Center and so many other "experiments," where the public was told there is nothing to worry about. Or will the risks be accepted, just as we accept the risks of driving a car? (Cars kill more than 30,000 Americans each year.) Will the public be allowed an informed choice?

For years to come we'll continue to see environmental refugees seeking a better and safer life in the Southwest, or wherever they can. Perhaps, in the distant future, historians will write about the plight of environmentally ill patients, just as books have been written about the tuberculosis migrations. The historians might write about the houses we built, the living conditions some of us had to endure, the treatments, the controversies and all the rest. Hopefully they'll also be able to write that the illnesses became well understood and curable — or at least that society took steps to help those stricken and to limit the number of new cases.

Bibliography

House Construction and Renovation

Anderson, B et al., Pre-contamination of new gypsum wallboard with potentially harmful fungal species, *Indoor Air,* 2014.

Baker-Laporte, Paula, Erica Elliot, John Banta. *Prescriptions for a Healthy House, third edition.* Gabriola Island, BC: New Catalyst Books, 2014.

Bower, John. *The Healthy House: How to buy one, How to build one, How to cure a sick one, 4th edition.* Bloomington, IN: The Healthy House Institute, 2001.

_____. *Healthy House Building for the New Millennium: A Design and Construction Guide.* Bloomington, IN: The Healthy House Institute, 2000.

Chiras, Daniel D. *The Solar House: passive solar heating and cooling.* Vermont: Chelsea Green Publishing, 2002.

Garlington, Phil. *Rancho Costa Nada – The Dirt Cheap Desert Homestead.* Washington: Loompanics, 2003.

Hobbs, Angela. *The Sick House Survival Guide: Simple Steps to Healthier Homes.* Gabriola Island, BC: New Society, 2003.

Jenkins, Joseph. *The Humanure Handbook – a guide to composting human manure.* Grove City, Pennsylvania: Joseph Jenkins, Inc.

Kahn, Lloyd, Blair Allen and Julie Jones. *The Septic System Owner's Manuel.* Bolinas: Shelter Publications, 2000.

Ludwig, Art. *Oasis with Graywater: Choosing, Building, and Using Greywater Systems*. Santa Barbara: Oasis Design, 2006.

May, Jeffrey and Connie May. *The Mold Survival Guide: for your home and your health*. Baltimore & London: Johns Hopkins University Press, 2004.

Nash, George. *Do-It-Yourself Housebuilding*. New York: Sterling Publishing, 1995.

Rea, William J. *Optimum Environments for Optimum Health and Creativity – Designing and Building a Healthy Home or Office*. Dallas: Crown Press, 2002.

Riley, Karl. *Tracing EMFs in Building Wiring and Grounding, Third Edition, revised*. West Tisbury, MA: Karl Riley, 2012.

Scher, Les and Carol Scher. *Finding & Buying Your Place in the Country*. Chicago: Dearborn Financial Publishing, 2000.

Steinemann, Anne. Ten questions concerning green buildings and indoor air quality, *Building and Environment, 112, 351-358, 2017*

Thompson, Athena. *Homes that Heal and those that don't*. Gabriola Island, BC: New Society, 2004.

Tudhope, Hilton. *Home for Health: Creating a Sanctuary for Healing,* Dallas, TX: Build for Health Press, 2018.

Venolia, Carol. *Healing Environments: your guide to indoor well-being*. Berkeley: Celestial Arts, 1988.

Healthy Housing Web Sites

buildahealthyhouse.com
eiwellspring.org/saferhousing.html
greenhome.com

greenbuildingadvisor.com
healthybuilding.net
planetthrive.com
radon.com
reshelter.org

Environmental Illness (MCS/EHS), etc.

AESSRA. *Living with Chemical Sensitivities*. Ringwood, VIC, Australia: AESSRA, 2016.

Aron, Elaine. *The Highly Sensitive Person*. New York: Broadway Books, 1997.

_____. *The Highly Sensitive Person in Love*. New York: Broadway Books, 2001.

Ashford, Nicholas and Claudia Miller. *Chemical Exposures: Low Levels and High Stakes (Second Edition)*. New York, NY: Van Nostrand Reinhold, 1998.

Becker, Robert O. *Cross Currents: The Perils of Electropollution – The Promise of Electromedicine*. New York: Tarcher, 1990.

_____, and Gary Selden. *The Body Electric*. New York: Quill, 1985.

Bevington, Michael. *Electromagnetic Sensitivity and Electromagnetic Hypersensitivity – A Summary*. Great Britain: Capability Books, 2013.

Blank, Martin. *Overpowered: the dangers of electromagnetic radiation and what you can do about it*. New York: Seven Stories Press, 2014.

Crofton, Kerry. *A Wellness Guide for the Digital Age – With Safer-Tech Solutions for All Things Wired and Wireless*. United States: Global WellBeing Books, 2014.

Crumpler, Diana. *Prostituting Science: the psychologisation of MCS, CFS, and EHS for political gain.* Maryborough, VIC, Australia: Inkling Australia, 2014.

Dadd, Debra Lynn. *Home Safe Home: Creating a Healthy Home Environment by Reducing Exposure to Toxic Household Products.* New York: Tarcher/Penguin, 2004.

Evans, Jerry. *Chemical and Electric Hypersensitivity – A Sufferer's Memoir.* Jefferson, NC: McFarland, 2010. Also available from Arizona State Braille and Talking Book Library (book 5779, 2015).

Firstenberg, Arthur. *The Invisible Rainbow: A History of Electricity and Life.* Santa Fe, NM: AGB Press, 2017.

Geary, James. The Man Who Was Allergic to Radio Waves. *Popular Science*, February 2010.

Gibson, Pamela Reed. Unmet medical care needs in persons with multiple chemical sensitivity. *Journal of Nursing Education and Practice,* Vol 6, No 5, 75-83, 2016.

_____. *Multiple Chemical Sensitivity: a survival guide.* Virginia: Earthrive Books, 2006.

Gorman, Carolyn. *Less-Toxic Alternatives.* Plano, TX: Caleta Press, 2010.

Granlund-Lind, Rigmor, and John Lind. *Black on White: Voices and Witnesses about Electro-Hypersensitivity: The Swedish Experience.* Sala: Mimers Brunn, 2005.

Grenville, Kate. The *Case Against Fragrance.* Melbourne, Australia: Text Publishing, 2017.

Hobbs, Angela. *The Sick House Survival Guide: Simple Steps to Healthier Homes.* Gabriola Island, BC: New Society, 2003.

Ingram, Sharon. Summer camp for families with electrically sensitive children, eiwellspring.org, 2014.

Jensen, Thilde. *The Canaries.* LENA Publications, 2013.

Johnson, Alison. *Amputated Lives: coping with chemical sensitivity*. Brunswick, Maine: Cumberland Press, 2008.

Ladberg, Gunilla. *Forced to Disconnect: Electrohypersensitive Fugitives in Sweden*. Sweden: Gunilla Ladberg Pedagogik & Språk, 2010.

Lyndsey, Anna. *Girl in the Dark*. New York: Anchor Books, 2015.

McCampbell, Ann. *Multiple Chemical Sensitivity*. Belmont, CA: Environmental Health Connection, 2011.

Molot, John. *12,000 Canaries Can't Be Wrong*. Toronto: ECW Press, 2014.

Niemark, Jill. Allergic to Life. *Discover*, November 2013.

Nordstrom, Gunni. *The Invisible Disease*. New Alresford, Hampshire, UK: O Books, 2004.

Pall, Martin. *Explaining "Unexplained Illnesses."* Boca Raton, FL: CRC Press, 2007.

Philips, Alasdair and Jean Philips. *The Powerwatch Handbook: Simple ways to make you and your family safer*. London, UK: Piatkus, 2006.

Platt, Mary Frances. The New Refugees. *Ragged Edge*, March/April, 2003.

Randolph, Theron G and Ralph W. Moss. *An Alternative Approach to Allergies (Revised Edition)*. New York: Harper & Row, 1990.

Reinhold, Robert. When life is toxic, *New York Times Magazine*, Sept 16, 1990.

Singer, Katie. *An electronic silent spring: facing the dangers and creating safe limits*. Great Barrington, MA: Portal Books, 2014.

Vedenetra, Hermitra Elan*tra. *Silicone Injury – Memoir of a Life and a Spiritual Journey*. Bloomington, IN: Author House, 2013.

Zwillinger, Rhonda. *The Dispossessed*. Paulden, AZ: The Dispossessed Outreach Project, 1999.

Resistance to Accepting Health Effects

Alster, Norm. *Captured Agency;* Edmond J. Safra Center for Ethics, Harvard University, 2015.

Ashford, Nicholas and Claudia Miller. *Chemical Exposures: Low Levels and High Stakes (Second Edition).* New York: Van Nostrand Reinhold, 1998 (chapter 9).

Blank, Martin. *Overpowered: the dangers of electromagnetic radiation and what you can do about it.* New York: Seven Stories Press, 2014.

Boyd, I., G. J. Rubin and S. Wessely, Taking refuge from modernity: 21st century hermits, *Journal of Research in Social Medicine,* 105, 2012.

Carlo, George and Martin Schram. *Cell Phones: Invisible hazards in the wireless age,* New York: Carroll & Graf Publishers, 2001.

Castleman, Barry L. *Asbestosis: Medical and Legal Aspects, 4th edition*. Englewood Cliffs, NJ: Aspen Law and Business, 1996.

Davis, Devra. *Disconnect: the truth about cell phone radiation, what industry has done to hide it, and how to protect your family*. New York: Penguin, 2010.

Gibson, Pamela Reed. Unmet medical care needs in persons with multiple chemical sensitivity. *Journal of Nursing Education and Practice,* Vol 6, No 5, 75-83, 2016.

Groopman, Jerome. *How doctors think,* New York: Mariner Books, 2007.

Hardell, Lennart. World Health Organization, radiofrequency and health – a hard nut to crack, *International Journal of Oncology,* 2017.

Huss, Anke et al. Source of funding and results of studies of health effects of mobile phone use, *Environmental Health Perspectives,* January 2007.

McCampbell, Ann. Multiple Chemical Sensitivities Under Siege, *Townsend Letter,* January 2001.

McGarity, Thomas and Wendy Wagner. *Bending Science: How special interests corrupt public health research.* Cambridge, MA: Harvard University Press, 2008.

Michaels, David. *Doubt is their product: How industry's assault on science threatens your health,* New York: Oxford University Press, 2008.

Nelson, Eric and Mark Worth, Boeing to ill workers: It's all in your head, Washington *Free Press,* Feb-Mar, 1994.

Smith, Rick and Bruce Lourie. *Slow Death by Rubber Duck – The secret dangers of everyday things.* Berkeley, CA: Counterpoint, 2009.

Tuberculosis Migration to the Southwest

Jones, Billy M. *Health-Seekers in the Southwest, 1817-1900.* Norman, OK: University of Oklahoma Press, 1967.

Kravetz, Robert E., and Alex Jay Kimmelman. *Healthseekers in Arizona.* Phoenix, AZ: Academy of Medical Sciences of Maricopa Medical Society, 1998.

Sheridan, Thomas E. *Arizona – A History.* Tucson, AZ: University of Arizona Press, 1995.

Motion Pictures

Homesick: Living with multiple chemical sensitivities. Directed by Susan Abod. USA: Dual Power Productions, 2013. DVD.

Mobilize: A Film About Cell Phone Radiation. Directed by Kevin Kunze. USA: Disinformation/Kunze Productions, 2014. DVD.

Multiple Chemical Sensitivity: A Life-Altering Condition. Directed by Alison Johnson. USA: Johnson/Startzman Film, 2013. DVD.

Safe. Directed by Todd Haynes. USA: Columbia/Sony Pictures, 1999. DVD.

The Sensitives. Directed by Drew Xanthopoulos. USA: Normie Productions, 2017. DVD.

Where Can We Live? - about being electrosensitive. Directed by Helene Aastrup Samuels. Sweden: Eira Film, 2011. DVD.

Sound Recording

Palmer, Kim (singer-songwriter). *Songs from a porcelain trailer.* Canada: Paradigm Records, PR18-2, 1999. Compact disc.

Index

Index